A CLEAN BILL OF HEALTH

A CLEAN BILL OF HEALTH

RESTORING AMERICAN MEDICAL EXCEPTIONALISM

MYLES SAUNDERS M.D.

"A Clean Bill of Health"- RESTORING AMERICAN MEDICAL EXCEPTIONALISM
Myles Saunders, MD
Copyright © 2015 (Health Address Communications, 9903 Santa Monica Blvd Suite 576. Beverly Hills, CA. 90212)• Telephone (310) 487-5555 • Fax (310) 858-7162

E-mail: drmylessaunders@yahoo.com

ISBN-10: 0692373411
ISBN-13: 978-0-692-37341-5

Printed in the United States

EDITOR: Steve Reinberg • S_Reinberg@hacommunications.net
PROJECT MANAGER: John Peragine • info@osiris-papers.com
INTERIOR DESIGN: Glen Edelstein • glenede@gmail.com
COVER DESIGN: Glen Edelstein • glen@hudsonvalleybookdesign.com

CONTENTS

To my wife and son, with undying love.

PREFACE

Millions of Americans believe that our healthcare system is broken and needs to be repaired, but believe that the Affordable Care Act (ACA) is not the solution, only the beginning of a host of new problems. For over four decades, I have played a part in the American healthcare system and bring a unique perspective to its reform.

As I climbed the education ladder from medical student to resident in training, ultimately becoming a practicing physician, I worked with Primary Stakeholders in the healthcare system, patients and families, doctors, and other caregivers who constitute the intimate, front line participants in medical delivery. Later, I worked with Secondary Stakeholders, those who are essential in the healthcare system but do not directly deal with patient care, such as government agencies, hospital systems, pharmaceutical companies, and healthcare insurance companies. Ultimately, the more Peripheral Stakeholders--professional associations, research organizations, administrators of medical education, and training facilities became part of my professional world.

After almost two decades as a practicing physician, I entered the research and entrepreneurial arenas of the healthcare industry, inspired by a vision to provide innovative, Internet-related products and services with the potential to improve the quality of and access to medical care anywhere in the world, while lowering the costs of healthcare delivery. For over a decade in this role, I was exposed to novel groups of stakeholders including business people, corporate and patent attorneys, domestic government and non-government agencies, travel and hospitality services, foreign medical systems and Ministries of Health. In addition, I worked directly with patients, providers, and a wide range of stakeholders in healthcare systems in countries throughout the Asia-Pacific region. Each culture manifested different sensibilities, expectations, and family experiences with local healthcare systems. They also held individual religious and dietary customs, and encountered their own set of local and regional diseases. Each culture, harbored different levels of trust with new doctors regardless of how ill they or members of their families might be.

From these perspectives, I began a serious comparison of healthcare systems of other countries while on the ground in many developing countries throughout the Asia-Pacific region. What would be the impact on healthcare delivery, of innovations that I hoped to introduce? Would they be scalable enough to affect larger groups or populations? And, would compliance be achievable? These were among the important questions that needed to be asked during healthcare reform at home, as well.

Critically thinking about healthcare systems in those terms inevitably lead me to question the U.S. healthcare system that I had previously taken for granted. I instinctively knew the U.S. system as the best in the world. No system in the world stood anywhere near American medical delivery in terms of its modernization, availability of top tier medical specialists, or all-important high technology diagnostic imaging devices, computerized information systems, or non-invasive anti-cancer equipment.

How had its growth been managed through the years? Did our healthcare system act like other complex entities and undergo anticipated changes in its life cycle? If so, where in the cycle was our health system now, and did that have any bearing on the progression of its weaknesses. Was our healthcare system still growing? Evolving? Or, had it reached a point at which it had to be changed or risk being toppled under its own weight? In addition, the most important question dealt with government's role as the cause of healthcare's ills in America.

Several experiences were to influence me profoundly. On my first international business trip in 2002, I traveled to the Sultanate of Oman on the Persian Gulf at the request of then, Ambassador to the United Nations, H.E. Hunaina Sultan Ahmed Al Mughairy. Quite by chance, I had recently read a World Health Organization1 (WHO) publication that ranked the healthcare systems of each of its 191 member "states." Oman's healthcare system happened happened to have been ranked as number one in accessibility, and was ranked number eight overall. Notably, in that report, the U.S. healthcare system ranked a poor 37th overall. I was eager to see what a top ranked healthcare system in the world looked like, especially in comparison with the system I had grown up with. What I found was strikingly different from what I had expected. That experience lead to many of my important insights into the politics of global medicine and its effects on U.S. healthcare policy.

During my years of business travel to different parts of the globe, I began thinking about American healthcare in a new way. Was the U.S. healthcare system as good as I thought it was? Were its weaknesses a necessary part of its complexity and size, or was I wrong, and had its true faults been hiddenby the high-tech neuro-surgery I practiced in Los Angeles? Each healthcare system that I examined gave me a keener insight into the fundamental workings of the U.S. healthcare system.

That intellectual exercise might have meant little beyond my own edification had it not been for the thunderclouds that I viewed in the distance that ultimately became part of the real world landscape that we now know as the Affordable Care Act (ACA). One thing became clear: policy analysts and decision makers were arrogantly and brazenly deciding the fate of the American people even though they knew that a majority were satisfied with their own healthcare and were dissatisfied with the proposed solution.

I have written this book because we have been forced into a profound healthcare predicament by the ACA. In fact, we are already behind the curve. We can, however, still extricate ourselves from the radical transformation that the ACA imposes not only on our healthcare system, but also on our way of life. As stakeholders in a once exceptional healthcare system, we bear the responsibility to bring our ideas into the public arena in order to avoid having our freedoms taken from us by remaining silent.

RESOURCES

1. www.who.int

INTRODUCTION

It was no accident that the American medical delivery system was borne of exceptionalism.

The modern medical system we know today took root between 1890 and 1910 when a small group of pioneers in the biological and physical sciences were hired to devise new systems of medical education, to train post-graduate residents, to develop modern laboratory research methods, and design new approaches to medical care. While the system that they developed was not perfect, it would remain exceptional and unrivaled by all but a few regional Western medical centers.

Taking place at the Johns Hopkins Hospital and Medical School in Baltimore, the "Hopkins experiment" forever changed the way medicine would be practiced by applying a unique system of medical knowledge to patient care that would become our medical delivery system, consisting of doctors and other healthcare providers interacting with patients in crucial, therapeutic, doctor-patient relationships. That intimate human experience would remain the most effective conduit for communicating and caring for patients and their families despite whatever high-technology devices might be added to the mix, or how remote the patient might be geographically from the doctor (telemedicine). Preserving the adequate time, inclination, and skills to deliver healthcare to patients would remain the doctors' original intent, and must be recognized as such in any meaningful reform.

Most of us have encountered elements of healthcare delivery (doctors, nurses, and hospitals) but are unaware of the enormous supporting industries, organizations, and individuals that comprise the greater healthcare system, each with their own interests. They include federal, state, and local governments, along with their regulatory bureaucracies, hospital corporations, pharmaceutical interests (Big Pharma), the health insurance industry, medical device manufacturers, and the combined group of American employers who, in paying for health insurance for their employees, would become the overwhelming influence on the private health insurance industry.

The greater U.S. healthcare system had become enormous and uncontrollable.

Thus, in the lead-up to healthcare reform, we had the luxury of a superb, though imperfect, medical delivery system that was enveloped in an enormous extended healthcare system, too complex to assure optimal access to care for everyone, too disorganized to prevent a multitude of institutional and professional errors that resulted in death, disability and suffering, and a system too inefficient to control spending.

In developing the ACA, government officials and other decision makers chose to enact a comprehensive set of laws that best affirmed the worldview of the Progressive politicians that held power in 2010 when President Obama signed the law.

Architects of the ACA chose to ignore many of the lessons of history, just as they chose not to follow the wishes of their constituents, most of whom were satisfied with their healthcare. Yet most Americans recognized weaknesses in the system that needed to be reformed. Along with many experts, they believed that the ACA would move America in the wrong direction without solving our healthcare problems.

In 2010 the ACA became a "wholesale overhaul of the healthcare sector of the economy in a single, massive bill of 2,700-plus pages," according to Robert Moffit of the Heritage Foundation.[1]

And, when it finally could be analyzed through an objective lens, when we found out what was in it, Americans learned that our exceptional healthcare system had been dismantled, and replaced by an unworkable system, devoid of the freedoms that make up the American character. The federal government had exerted control over healthcare that extended to all aspects of medical practice, destined to turn the best medical care into an average one, at best.

This book is divided into three functional parts: Part One discusses the origins and unique characteristics of American medical exceptionalism. After setting the stage, in Chapter One, an eye-opening look at the heretofore mostly hidden intentions that lurk within President Barrack Obama's signature legislative accomplishment, in Chapter Two, I discuss how the same values that were exhibited by the Founding Fathers of our nation were adopted by an assemblage of some of the most unique, gifted, physicians and scientists who created a modern, experimental healthcare system that was rightly dubbed American medical exceptionalism. Chapter Three connects the "Judeo-Christian values" that form the foundation of America's first principles as stated in the Declaration of Independence and U.S. Constitution, with their part in developing a set of bio-ethical guidelines to be followed by all stakeholders who participate in the U.S. healthcare system.

Part Two of the book deals with U.S. healthcare in the 20th Century, leading up to the passage of the ACA in 2010. Chapters Four and Five answer the questions of just how good the U.S. Medical Delivery System was, and what reasons underlay growing negative perceptions by Americans as well as 'citizens of the world.' It is now well known that its' reputation was tarnished due to a campaign of disinformation to disparage and unduly criticize the U.S. healthcare system. The book deals with the serious propaganda campaign waged against U.S. healthcare, revealing who perpetrated this scheme, how they did it, and most importantly, why. The effect of that campaign so unfairly lead to the disparagement of the

U.S. healthcare system by global entities such as the World Health Organization, that its "critics became useful tools used persuasively by President Obama to advance his stated plan to move America toward a collectivist, single-payer healthcare system."[2] And still, as these chapters show, that when measured head-to-head with the collectivist Nationalized Healthcare systems in Canada, the UK, and Western Europe, the U.S. healthcare system prior to the ACA could be demonstrated to perform better. And, I will include the outcome of my in-country analysis of Oman's healthcare system. In Chapter Six, I describe the major "moving parts" of healthcare systems that are subject to healthcare reform, including unique characteristics of and challenges to the U.S. healthcare reform. Chapter Seven deals with the impact of the ACA on healthcare in the U.S. and its impingement on our freedoms and way of life. From there, in Part Three, I will show that there is a better way to make the much-needed healthcare reforms based upon established best practices, and the first principles of our nation.

In Chapter Eight, I discuss how the Federal government has repudiated the core, or, first principles of our country that the Founding Fathers expressed in the Declaration of Independence and U.S. Constitution. Only by lessening government's intrusion on the business of the people can we restore those freedoms that originally gave us American exceptionalism and American medical exceptionalism.

Chapter Nine, deals with one of the most important manifestations of our first principles, the morality of working within the system of capitalism and the free market, and how that creates the road to restoration of our healthcare system.

REFERENCES

1. Moffit,Reforming Health Care on the Foundation of First Principles(2), Robert E. Moffit, Ph.D., a Senior Fellow in the Center for Policy Innovation at The Heritage Foundation.

2. Atlas, Scott W. (2012-01-03). In Excellent Health: Setting the Record Straight on America's Health Care (Hoover Institution Press Publication) (Kindle Locations 3448-3450). Chicago Distribution. Kindle Edition. Atlas, Scott W. (2012-01-03).

CHAPTER ONE

"LIKE STRAY CATS AND DOGS..."

As President Barack Obama pushed for a new federal health law, the largest reform to healthcare[1] since Medicare in 1965, he made a simple, often repeated pledge to the American people: "If you like your insurance plan, you can keep your plan." And, there was a second half to the President's promise: "No matter how we reform healthcare," Obama said in 2009, "we will keep this promise: if you like your doctor, you will be able to keep your doctor.[2] But, what was to become known in 2013 as the "Lie-of-the-Year," [3] barely hinted at the deception that the President knew had been written into the ACA years before.

Over the years, the President had openly made his wishes known to his valued Progressive constituencies: "I happen to be a proponent of a single-payer health care plan"[4] and, referring to a possible lag period before a single-payer plan could be enacted: "There's going to be potentially some transition process. I can envision a decade out or 15 years or 20 years out [sic]," Obama said. We now know that it was never his intention to wait, according to Kerry Picket of Breitbart news. [5] However, the President knew that if his true intentions were known at the time, the ACA would never become law.

In reality, the bill that would later become the Patient Protection and Affordable Care Act (PPACA, or, ACA), contained a deceptive mechanism that would force a single-payer system on the American people almost immediately, against their wishes, as reported by Andrew McCarthy in the National Review.[4] McCarthy went on to say that the scheme would be put into motion upon signing the new bill into law. [6] But until then, the President and top administration officials had to keep up their well-known lies. Thirty-seven times they repeated their lies until they were forced to admit to it due to the HealthCare.gov website debacle.

In October, 2013, after almost five years of lead-time, and at least five-hundred million dollars in taxpayer funding, the ACA opened for business in the form of the HealthCare.gov website. For the first time, eligible consumers could enroll online in the new health insurance system. The website's roll-out, however, proved disastrous as users were subjected to inordinately long wait times, errors, bugs, and other problems.[6] The ACA health insurance exchange fiasco revealed that 4 million people who were in the individual health insurance market had lost their insurance policies, and were forced to purchase more expensive ACA plans through the online exchanges.[7] Another 10 million people in the individual market were also at risk for losing their policies, and being forced into purchasing an ACA policy. For many, this first experience with the workings of the ACA was a foreshadowing of the government's inability to effectively run healthcare. But for President Obama, these events forced a public apology to something he knew all along would be coming.

However, there was more deception to come. In November 2013 the healthcare policy expert, Avik Roy, wrote an article in Forbes Magazine online which carried the headline, "Obama Officials In 2010: 93 Million Americans Will Be Unable to Keep Their Health Plans under Obamacare." Not only those in the individual market, but also those in the market for employer-sponsored health insurance were due to lose their plans.[8] "The Obama administration had known for three years that when the employer mandate was to be implemented in 2015, after a delay of a year, up to 93 million additional Americans would be forced out of their employer-sponsored health insurance plans." It was only by delaying the Employer mandate until 2015 for businesses with 100 employees or more, and to 2016, two years longer than originally envisioned under the Affordable Care Act,[9] for businesses with from 50-99 employees, that President Obama was able to keep the lid on this bombshell. [10]

It always stood to reason that most or all of consumers seeking private insurance would eventually have to purchase policies through the exchanges that were being set up by the ACA, Avik Roy explains, since premiums from policies purchased by this large pool of patients, who, in general, tended to be in good health, and hence tended to under-utilize the healthcare system, were necessary to pay for seniors and low income consumers who use healthcare services the most. [11,12] In other words, it was essential that "young healthy people...buy overpriced, largely superfluous coverage to underwrite the cost of insuring older and sicker people," Roy reports. [13,14]

Despite the promise made by President Obama, that people could keep their old policies, that they would be 'grandfathered' in, or exempted from the new rules set up by the ACA, "subsequent regulations from the Obama administration interpreted that provision so narrowly as to prevent most plans from gaining this protection," according to NBC's Lisa Myers, as reported in the Roy article.[8,13] In reality, the ACA demanded that all Americans purchase health insurance, whether they want it or not, and very few existing plans fit the description necessary to be exempted, forcing most people to buy entirely different policies that offered services that most Americans "don't need, don't want, and won't use, for a higher price."

This closely guarded secret -- that virtually no plans would be 'grandfathered' because "they did not meet the health law's changing definition of compatible," had been policy even before the President made his famous promise, and had existed in plain sight, for anyone to see in the June 2010 Federal Register. Avik Roy of Forbes online further reported that "administration officials predicted massive disruption of the private insurance market" if this news became widespread. So, in order to keep the ACA on track, President Obama had to lie and say that people could keep their own insurance while the predicted "massive disruption of the private insurance market" was soon to be exploited in the administration's plan to takeover healthcare altogether.

As part of the massive collectivist system the Obama administration was about to foist on the nation, there was another "whopper" [15,16] also hidden in plain sight in the Federal Register. According to former New York Lieutenant Governor, Betsy McCaughey, a healthcare journalist and critic, the ACA was tightening the federal government's grip over your doctor — even if you're paying for private insurance, and despite President Obama's often repeated pledge to the contrary.[17] According to McCaughey, "Beginning in 2015, insurance companies will be barred from doing business with doctors who fail to comply with the evolving rules being written in the name of ensuring 'health-care quality,' which of course could mean anything." The ACA contained the expressed powers to compel unimagined regulations on doctors and medical practices that could, for example, destroy the time honored doctor-patient relationship.

Ironically, it was in a lecture given to the gathered House Republicans in Baltimore (January, 2010), that President Obama telegraphed the ACA's hidden agenda. He conceded, as reported by Kerry Picket of the Washington Times, "If you look at the package that we presented, and there are some stray cats and dogs that got in there that we were eliminating...we were in the process of eliminating....I think that some of the provisions that got snuck [sic] in might have violated the pledge, and so we were in the process of scrubbing this [sic] and making sure that it was tight." [17,18] However, not all of the "stray cats and dogs" were eliminated.

Although multiple reports had been published warning of its inevitability, it took Andrew C. McCarthy III, a former Assistant United States Attorney for the Southern District of New York, the leader of the team that successfully prosecuted the terrorists behind the first World Trade Tower bombing in 1995, to fully illuminate the Presidents "scheme." [19 20 21 22]

As the President apologized to the American people for the "Lie-of-the-Year" in November 2013, McCarthy points out, he knew that the bill "pushes all Americans into government markets, dictates the content of the "private" insurance product; sets the price; micromanages patient access, business practices, and fees of doctors; and rations medical care," all of which sow "a financing crisis into the system, designed to explode after the Leviathan has so enveloped health care, and so decimated the private medical sector, that a British- or Canadian-style 'free' system — formerly unthinkable for the United States — becomes the inexorable solution."[23 24]

The ACA had been a multi-layered deception all along, made possible by a total lack of transparency, an advantage taken by two key participants in the Obamacare scheme. First, the Speaker of the House of Representatives, Nancy Pelosi, famously said on March 9, 2010, that all would be revealed in time, but for now, just days before President Obama was to sign the bill into law: "We have to pass the bill so you can find out what is in it." [25 26]

Second, the Obamacare 'house of cards' had been purposely hidden from the public according to a chief architect of the ACA, MIT Economics Professor, Jonathan Gruber: "...that lack of transparency was a major part of getting Obamacare passed because 'the stupidity of the American voter' would have killed the law if more people knew what was in it," in a tape of a 2013 panel discussion, reported by Avik Roy. Gruber went on to explain that he had to construct a complex system of insurance regulations within the law in order to conceal from voters that the ACA really was a huge redistribution of wealth from the young and healthy to the old and unhealthy, and, that if Democrats had been honest about these facts, including that the law's individual mandate was, in effect, a major tax hike, the ACA would never have passed Congress.[27][28]

Since being signed into law, the ACA has sharply split Americans along party lines, largely because of the secretive nature of what was known about it. However, by November, 2014, as negative news about the ACA's impact emerged almost daily, it became clear that we were far worse off than before as the law eroded our once excellent healthcare system as government intrusion grew under the new healthcare law. The 2014 midterm elections resulted in a Republican wave, and as the party regained a majority in the Senate and widened its majority in the House of Representatives. President Obama's approval rating stood at 40 percent -- the lowest recorded during his six years in office.[29]

This set the stage for Americans to solidify their opinions behind their disapproval of the ACA.

But what, if anything, could be done to rectify the situation? The answer comes from the Declaration of Independence and the U.S. Constitution -- the sources of our "first principles". Since the government derives its power "from the consent of the governed," Thomas Jefferson wrote in the preamble to the Declaration, when it becomes destructive of our unalienable rights of life, liberty and the pursuit of happiness, the people have the right "to alter or to abolish it, and to institute new Government." In this case, it means we have to change healthcare reform. To do this, we shall almost certainly have to change the government leadership through elections.

How did we ever get to this dangerous tipping point? How did we replace the greatest healthcare system in the world with an unworkable, quasi-collectivist, near single-payer scheme? And how do we restore our great healthcare system? The answer can be found in the legacy left to us by America's Founding Fathers, as well as the founders of our healthcare system.

In the upcoming pages, I will answer those questions, and address as well: What were the origins of American Medical exceptionalism, and how did a perfect political storm cause its demise? How did the struggle to restore medical exceptionalism take on global proportions? And most importantly, how do our first principles lead us to restore our great healthcare, and what will that system look like?

REFERENCES:

1   Style note: Is it healthcare, health-care, or health care? I have chosen to use the single, non-hyphenated form of the word, both as a noun (Healthcare must be reformed) and adjective (I agree with healthcare professionals), consistently, throughout this book, unless quoting a source that takes a different spelling. Comparing authoritative sources, I have found some that opine that the one word version is taking over in the English speaking world (http://grammarist.com/spelling/healthcare/), some that insist that the compound word be hyphenated, (http://www.chicagomanualofstyle.org/qanda/data/faq/topics/Compounds.html) and still others that call for two separate words, differentiating between its use as a noun or adjective. I chose to remain consistent with the compound word both for simplicity and easy readability, as well as for efficacy in search engine use on the Internet.

2   http://swampland.time.com/2013/11/19/you-can-keep-your-doctor-obamacares-next-broken-promise/

3   http://www.politifact.com/truth-o-meter/article/2013/dec/12/lie-year-if-you-like-your-health-care-plan-keep-it/

4   Remarks to AFL – CIO in Flashback: Obama's Campaign to Transition to Single Payer Health Care (VIDEO), 'The Conversation," KERRY PICKET 29 Oct 2013, http://www.breitbart.com/InstaBlog/2013/10/29/Flashback-Obama-s-Campaign-to-Transition-to-Single-Payer-Health-Care-VIDEO

5   Obama - (SEIU Healthcare Forum) – 3/24/07 in Flashback: Obama's Campaign to Transition to Single Payer Health Care (VIDEO), 'The Conversation," KERRY PICKET 29 Oct 2013,http://www.breitbart.com/ InstaBlog/2013/10/29/Flashback-Obama-s-Campaign-to-Transition-to-Single-Payer-Health-Care-VIDEO

6   U.S. House of Representatives Committee on Oversight and Government Reform Darrell Issa (CA-49), Chairman http://oversight.house.gov/ wp-content/uploads/2014/09/Healthcare-gov-Report-Final-9-17-14.pdf

7   http://www.healthbeatblog.com/2014/02/did-president-obama-lie-when-he-said-if-you-like-the-policy-you-have-you-can-keep-it-context-is-everything/

8   http://www.forbes.com/sites/theapothecary/2013/10/31/obama-officials-in-2010-93-million-americans-will-be-unable-to-keep-their-health-plans-under-obamacare/

9   http://www.washingtonpost.com/national/health-science/white-house-delays-health-insurance-mandate-for-medium-sized-employers-until-2016/2014/02/10/ade6b344-9279-11e3-84e1-27626c5ef5fb_story.html

10   The Affordable Care Act: An Update on the Employer Mandate William A. Dombi, Esq. MARCH ON WASHINGTON Conference & Exposition March 24, 2014 http://www.nahc.org/assets/1/7/MoW14-104.pdf

11   http://www.nihcm.org/pdf/DataBrief3%20Final.pdf

12   Avik Roy, Forbes, http://www.forbes.com/sites/theapothecary/2013/10/31/ obama-officials-in-2010-93-million-americans-will-be-unable-to-keep-their-health-plans-under-obamacare/requirements

13   Ibid, Avik Roy

14   http://www.washingtonpost.com/blogs/wonkblog/wp/2013/10/29/this-is-why-obamacare-is-cancelling-some-peoples-insurance-plans/

15   ObamaCare's latest whopper from nypost.com January 1, 2014 https:// www.instapaper.com/read/52272367

16   http://nypost.com/2014/01/01/obamacares-latest-whopper/ Betsy Mccaughey's

17   The ACA has "snuck" Obama: Health Care Bill "Might Have Violated Pledge" On Keeping Some Doctors And Insurers, January 29, 2010,(http://www.realclearpolitics.com/video/2010/01/29/obama_health_

care_bill_might_have_violated_pledge_on_keeping_some_doctors_and_insurers.html)

18   http://www.washingtontimes.com/blog/watercooler/2010/jan/31/videoobama-health-care-bill-some-provisions-got-sn/#ixzz3IbNmoiCV

19   Andrew C. McCarthy The Scheme behind the Obamacare Fraud, October 3, 2014, National Review Online http://www.nationalreview.com/article/364667/scheme-behind-obamacare-fraud-andrew-c-mccarthy

20   Obama admin. knew millions could not keep their health insurance - NBC News nbcnews.com

21   October 28, 2013 Obama Officials In 2010: 93 Million Americans Will Be Unable To Keep Their Health Plans Under Obamacare.

22   Forbes http://www.forbes.com/sites/theapothecary/2013/10/31/obama-officials-in-2010-93-million-americans-will-be-unable-to-keep-their-health-plans-under-obamacare/ October 3, 2014 at 06:57AM

23   DOJ: Majority Will Lose Employer-Based Healthcare Once Obamacare's Employer Mandate Kicks In pjmedia.com · November 18, 2013

24   Scheme behind the Obamacare Fraud National Review Online· by Andrew C. McCarthy, November 23, 2013

25   http://dailysignal.com/2010/03/10/video-of-the-week-we-have-to-pass-the-bill-so-you-can-find-out-what-is-in-it/

26   http://en.wikiquote.org/wiki/Nancy_Pelosi

27   http://www.forbes.com/sites/theapothecary/2014/11/10/aca-architect-the-stupidity-of-the-american-voter-led-us-to-hide-obamacares-tax-hikes-and-subsidies-from-the-public/

28   http://www.forbes.com/sites/theapothecary/2012/03/22/how-obamacare-dramatically-increases-the-cost-of-insurance-for-young-workers/

29   http://www.washingtonpost.com/politics/poll-shows-obama-approval-low-gop-enthusiasm-higher-than-democrats/2014/10/14/d9e7e4d6-53d5-11e4-ba4b-f6333e2c0453_story.html

CHAPTER TWO:

FIRST PRINCIPLES & AMERICAN MEDICAL EXCEPTIONALISM

"[A] GOLDEN thread has run throughout the history of the world, consecutive and continuous, the work of the best men in successive ages. From point to point it still runs, and when near, you feel it as the clear and bright and searchingly irresistible light, which Truth throws forth when great minds conceive it."

- WILLIAM OSLER, MD[1]

A NEW ORDER OF THE AGES

It had been over a decade since the Founding Fathers had written and signed the Declaration of Independence. (1776) The newly declared independent nation had won its liberty and the Framers had written and signed a new Constitution. (1787) And, even as they awaited ratification of the first ten amendments, known as the Bill of Rights (1791), they knew that they had entered into "an experiment in governance unlike any in history."[2] As social scientist and author, Charles Murray discusses in his book, "American Exceptionalism, An Experiment in History,"[2] the Founders certainly believed that they were creating something of extraordinary significance. That's why, according to Murray, they changed the motto on the Great Seal of the United States, to novus ordo seclorum—"a new order of the ages." There could be no doubt that our new nation was "exceptional, with political and civic cultures that had no counterparts anywhere else."[2]

The United States was founded by men with some of the best minds and foresight in history. They brought together philosophy of enlightenment figures like John Locke and Baron de Montesquieu, along with their own knowledge of classical philosophies,[3,4] religious beliefs and understanding of human nature. Rejecting the oppression of the past, these men embarked on an experiment to create a constitutional republic with foundational, or, first principles that would secure our freedom and liberty.[5,6] Thomas Jefferson saw in these principles, self-evident truths that he incorporated into the Declaration of Independence, which became our moral and ethical guide, and through James Madison and other Framers, the U.S. Constitution "became the living embodiment of a government [our laws] based on these First Principles."[5]

WHAT ARE THE FIRST PRINCIPLES?

The first principles[5] of our nation are those core premises upon which our country was founded. The Declaration of Independence and U.S. Constitution are the extant sources of those principles:

Rule of Law - The law governs everyone.
Unalienable Rights - Everyone is naturally endowed by their Creator with certain rights (Rights come from God, not government).
Equality - All persons are created equal under the law.

Social Compact - Governments are instituted by the people and derive their just powers from the consent of the governed

Limited Government - Government must be strong enough to fulfill its legitimate purposes as stated in the Constitution, yet protect our unalienable rights.

Private Property Rights - The Founders believed private property rights were intertwined with liberty.

Right to Declare Revolution - when the other First Principles are being infringed by the government.

All of the countless ethical and legal principles to which we adhere are derived from first principles, the only self-evident truths. They are the axioms, while all other principles that follow are corollaries.

This unique combination of political, intellectual, and religious heritage[6] resulted in 'American exceptionalism'. "This new spirit of exceptionalism became an energizing and uniting characteristic of the American ethos,"[6] as journalist, Patrick Buchanan put it. This same spirit can be shown to also be integral to American medical exceptionalism.

One hundred years after the founding of our nation, another small group of exceptional men and women, energized by that same ethos, met in Baltimore where they were recruited based on their unusual expertise and experience in the biological and physical sciences. They were charged to develop an innovative, experimental healthcare model for a new university and medical school, amply funded, with a $6 million gift from the railroad and real estate magnate, Johns Hopkins.[7] This group forged the model for what was to become the best healthcare delivery system in the world, and what has been called before and after American medical exceptionalism.[10] Thus, a common bond of exceptionalism was formed between the founding of a new country, and the formation of a new medical system, both derived from first principles acting as guideposts, indicating the best practices with which to carry them out and preserve them through reform.

As citizens, we are not only obligated to understand and adhere to the first principles, but we must also recognize these principles as the source of our exceptionalism. As practitioners and potential reformers, we recognize that healthcare exceptionalism further requires that we do our best to deliver healthcare's first intent of diagnosis, treatment and prevention of disease, and to enter into trusting relationships with our patients, inculcating the knowledge that each is receiving the best care in the world -- guided by the first principles of individualism and the right to life.[8] Unlike any provision found in the ACA, our reforms will elevate and restore healthcare to exceptionalism by placing our patients in the center of the healthcare decision making process (principles of autonomy[9] and healthcare freedom), and by empowering them with economic liberty (principle of the right to property).*

AMERICAN MEDICINE FROM LATE-NINETEENTH CENTURY

With the advent of the remarkable Johns Hopkins University and Hospital staff, modern medicine took root between 1890 and 1910 during what would later be looked upon as the great Hopkins Experiment. For the first time, according to both his vision and purpose of endowment, Johns Hopkins, himself, deemed that the hospital would form part of the medical school, combining laboratory research with bedside teaching, thereby emphasizing the goal of "advancing, rather than merely transmitting, knowledge."[11]

Before 1890 doctors had surprisingly little to learn, describes author Ira Rutkow in his book, Seeking the Cure: A History of Medicine in America. [12] They could be looked upon as solitary practitioners who simply followed the untested theories of their mentors. The few existing U.S. medical schools required only a high school diploma, or less, for admission. The science of medicine was also in its infancy. Germ theory did not even come into existence until 1861 with the work of Louis Pasteur, and Robert Koch in Europe.[11]

Medical care was in constant flux. Despite the fact that it had long been recognized that many patients got better by themselves, with the first signs of illness, doctors almost always undertook intensive medical intervention in the form of draining off fluids, for without it, so they thought, illnesses would certainly worsen and lead to death. And if a doctor recommended only rest and quiet, augmented perhaps by rudimentary sedatives or laxatives, questions invariably arose whether he was doing enough. Doctors were smug with their advice, and became even more disconcerting when questioned regarding their prowess.[11]

This was also the age before adequate anesthesia was available, nor was it known that infections were caused by lack of hygiene. Thus, surgeons were forced to perform operations without effective anesthesia or hygienic technique. In order to perform even the most rudimentary operation, surgeons relied on assistants to hold the unfortunate patient down while they operated as fast as possible, trying to minimize infection and pain before the patient passed out from shock.[11]

AMERICAN MEDICAL EXCEPTIONALISM AND FIRST PRINCIPLES

The Hopkins experience changed all that. Scientific and ethical (first) principles elevated healthcare to new standards. New thinking drove patient care toward a greater use of the scientific method as well as toward patient-centeredness, where patients, not the doctors, became the main focus of attention (principles of patient autonomy derived from individualism). Doctors began sharing ethical responsibilities with patients according to a new social contract that defined the doctor-patient relationship more clearly than ever.

Even today, virtually everyone is touched by the founders of modern American medicine. The men and women who created the finest medical delivery system ever seen were part of a long tradition that mirrored the transformation of the country from the days of the horse and buggy to those of the moon landing and beyond. However, it was not the unrivaled technical achievements of these pioneers of medicine and the space program that made America or American medicine, exceptional. Rather, it was the highest standards of science, combined with ethical precepts of America's first principles.

And, it is precisely this vital combination that we are in danger of losing under our current healthcare reform which nullifies proven principles, and goes a long way to eliminate two defining attributes of American medicine that have set us apart from every other healthcare system in the world, and are derived from freedoms enunciated in our first principles: the freedom for patients to benefit from investment in high-tech bio-medical research not curtailed by government (principle of limited government), and for individual patients to have the best care in the world by the best medical specialists (principles of individualism and healthcare freedom). These critical elements derive their legitimacy from America's first principles, and by de-emphasizing them, as is done by the ACA, healthcare reform moves U.S. healthcare in the wrong direction, toward collectivism.

Maintaining American medical exceptionalism has never been guaranteed. It requires ongoing commitments to constant reform by building on its strengths and not, as some critics have called for, dismantling them with no proven, effective replacement. The ability to improve without destroying is the true test of exceptionalism.

EXCEPTIONALISM AND THE FATHER OF MODERN MEDICINE

In the summer of 1897, the Reverend Frederick Gates decided he would use his summer vacation to bone up on medicine. A medical student friend recommended "The Principles and Practice of Medicine," by William Osler. The textbook was at that time one of a kind. Published in 1892, it was the first great textbook of modern medicine. It was at once a monument of nineteenth century medicine and a precursor to the twentieth century.[13] Gates found the book "one of the most intensely interesting he had ever read," but was "amazed at how few diseases could be treated effectively." As Osler biographer, Michael Bliss, discusses, [13] Gates realized that with the infusion of philanthropy, medicine might extend its reaches and methods, progressing to more of an exact science that would greatly benefit the country and the world. Gates held the unique position as philanthropic adviser to the oil magnate, John D. Rockefeller, and one of his jobs was to recommend worthy causes to fund. At the same time, Gates learned of a remarkable group of researchers and clinicians in Baltimore that included Osler whom he highly recommended to Rockefeller as worthy of support. It was through the patronage of Frederick Gates that John D. Rockefeller, inspired by the enlightened medical vision of William Osler, established the renowned scientific research center, the Rockefeller Institute.

Osler was later to be recognized as the Father of Modern Medicine -- this without ever making any great scientific breakthroughs. [13] However, Osler's contribution to American medicine would be exceptional.

William Osler, became the head of the team that had essentially 'invented' modern American medicine." More than just "the greatest physician of his time," Osler, was an accomplished classical scholar who celebrated "The Golden thread," [1] our common medical lineage, using the discoveries and breakthroughs of all who came before him. "[13] His sense of history and reverence for the traditions of the past were likewise transmitted to those that came after him. Osler was to create a culture of learning that carried through to the new American medical system "blend[ing] the art and science of medicine perhaps better than anyone else."[14] He promulgated the ethic of working and studying hard as a role model of Judeo-Christian values from which our first principles are derived.

Born, raised, and educated in Canada, Osler was awarded a hereditary title of Baronet by the British Crown and made Regius Professor of Medicine at Oxford University later in his life. His biographer, Michael Bliss said, that Osler was "an observer and scholar, a teacher of the natural history of disease," reported on the characteristics, diagnosis, and treatment of an amazing variety of diseases, syndromes, and cases. "Osler's revolutionary impact as a teacher, was to create, in concert with other expert Hopkins staff members, the clinician-scientist, a new type of hybrid physician who was to become instrumental in producing most of the major achievements and progress in medicine, generation-after-generation to the present time."[13]

FROM EXCEPTIONAL TO EXCEPTIONALISM

The ability to track the progress of medical history from epoch to epoch through the imagination of William Osler, became a useful tool in helping physicians maintain an "unbroken lineage" with what our ancestors considered essential principles. These were the methods by which they arrived at their conclusions, and we use them to determine whether information is still relevant today. Osler believed that, on balance, the progress of medicine has been spectacular, that modern health care offers one of the finest examples of the possibility of "man's redemption of man."[13]

By incorporating principles from the past, some relatively recent, and some ancient, Osler began to transform the medical profession from a trade into a profession. To make physicians more professional, Osler felt that a standardized, high-level pre-medical education was required. From that point forward, a college degree became a requirement to enter medical school. That was just the beginning.

The Hopkins experiment was about to revolutionize medical education, the practice of medicine, and medical research,[14] by creating the template for what was to become the most successful model of academic medicine of all times. Hopkins recruited, world-class physicians and scientists who were to become full-time chiefs of their respective services. Each, whether primarily a laboratory researcher, or a clinician who primarily managed patient care, would have unprecedented laboratory facilities that were located close to the hospital wards. As staff members, they would each have a full-time salary, freeing them to utilize their time as they chose, between teaching students on the wards, or conducting research in their nearby laboratory. Medical research by both faculty and students was fostered as integral to the educational process, the consequences of which became a Johns Hopkins hallmark, and the basis for American medical exceptionalism for over a century to follow: the clinician-scientist [13][14]

The insight to foster physicians to conduct laboratory research programs while performing the responsibilities of patient care lead to the unprecedented ability to discover causes of diseases, as well as practice new approaches to treatment.[13]

Under the direction of William Osler and his associates, the training of new doctors was revolutionized. Osler introduced the practice of bedside teaching of medical students. By making rounds with a handful of students, he was able to first demonstrate a given technique, and then have students learn it by doing. In that manner, students learned to take medical histories through proper doctor-patient interviews, and to perform thorough physical examinations. [13][14]

By teaching the art of practicing medicine in this way, to not only medical students, but also graduate physicians, a new system was developed that produced specialists, physicians who have undergone advanced training in order to become expert in a specific area of medicine.

Osler named that new system "residency" as he believed that in order to adequately prepare physicians for the rigors of medical practice, newly graduated doctors should spend most of their time, in the hospital, training in their craft. This was the beginning of the full-time, sleep-in residency[13] that so characterized doctors' specialty training thereafter. Doctors might spend up to eight years training in that restricted, hospital environment as they worked their way up a competitive pyramid that included multiple first year interns, up to a hard-won, single Chief Resident at the end of their training. By acting as part of the treating staff from the beginning, the higher they ascended, the more they assumed responsibility for direct patient care.

Osler's closest friend and colleague at Hopkins, the great neurosurgeon, Harvey Cushing, became the first product of the vision held by Osler and his group. Becoming a world leader in neurosurgery, Cushing stands as but one example of the exceptionalism that the Hopkins system would repeatedly produce and send out to perpetuate the system throughout their distinguished careers.

A LESSON FOR HEALTHCARE REFORM

Our nation and the nation's medical care system share the same roots. In addition, these principals must become the bedrock of healthcare reform. Robert Moffit, Director of the Center for Health Policy Studies at the Heritage Foundation, points out, "Just as most political discussions in the United States, the healthcare debate has turned into a debate about the size and scope of federal power. Healthcare reform must not only address the problems of cost, quality, and access, but also proceed in accordance with the Constitution and enlist the proper authorities of state and national government in their respective spheres."[15]

This admonition originated early in the course of America's healthcare debate. Dr. Benjamin Rush, a physician and signer of the Declaration of Independence, argued for two additional individual freedoms: the right to the freedom of medicine and the individual's right to choose his or her care in a free and open fashion. Rush warned of the day when medicine could and would be controlled by a single organization. Just as the great French political commentator, Alexis de Tocqueville, was later to warn of a soft-despotism,[2] the power of government to, in a manner resembling parental authority, attempt to keep people "in perpetual childhood" by relieving them "from all the trouble of thinking and all the cares of living, Rush and the other physicians at the convention[16] understood the possibility of medical despotism.

As medicine became more grounded in science and therefore driven by repeatable, observationally proven outcomes, it was important that reason, science, liberty, and enlightenment be allowed to become the framework of modern medical exceptionalism. Rush would not allow medicine to become restrained by the self-serving interests of the church, governments, or worse, the egocentric, self-serving doctors and scientists linked to the political despots of the time.

REFERENCES:

1   Sir William Osler (Walter Moxon, Pilocereus Senilis and Other Papers, 1887. Cited by Sir William Osler- The Evolution of Modern Medicine a Series of Lectures Delivered at Yale University on the Silliman Foundation in April, 1913 (Kindle Locations 36-37).) (Kindle Edition)

2   American Exceptionalism: An Experiment in History (Values and Capitalism) by Charles Murray location 19, 51}

3   http://en.wikipedia.org/wiki/Thomas_Jefferson_and_education#Views_on_classical_learning

4   http://www.history.ac.uk/reviews/review/1285

5   http://www.americassurvivalguide.com/americas-first-principles.php

6   American exceptionalism · by Patrick Joseph Buchanan · Wikipedia, the free encyclopedia en.wikipedia.org February 15, 2007

7   The History of Johns Hopkins Medicine, http://www.hopkinsmedicine.org/about/history/

8   http://iantyrrell.wordpress.com/papers-and-comments/

9   http://www.hhs.gov/ohrp/humansubjects/guidance/belmont.html

*   Throughout this book I refer to the four principles of medical ethics, taken from the Belmont Report of The National Commission for the Protection of Human Subjects of Biomedical and Behavioral Research (1974) 9 as discussed in AMA Journal of Ethics10 "Modern medical ethics has been tremendously influenced, both in theory and in practice, by the four principles approach to bioethics, which was generally developed from the 1978 "Belmont Report" and the work of Thomas Beauchamp and James Childress. According to these models, a physician's moral ob-

ligation toward his or her patient is defined by four ethical principles—respect for autonomy, nonmaleficence, beneficence, and justice. Respect for autonomy dictates that patients who have decision-making capacity have a right to voice their medical treatment preferences, and physicians have the concomitant duty to respect those preferences. Non-maleficence directs physicians to maximize the benefit to patients while minimizing the harm. Beneficence promotes the welfare and best interest of patients. Finally, justice demands fair, equitable, and appropriate treatment for all patients. These ethical principles are commonly referred to in professional ethical guidelines and applied in clinical decision-making.

10   http://journalofethics.ama-assn.org/2008/03/msoc1-0803.html

11   A Model of Its Kind, McGeehee et al, JAMA, June 2, 1969—Vol 261, No, 21 http://dcs.jhmi.edu/cvo/AModelOfItsKind.pdf

12   Rutkow, Ira (2010-03-27). Seeking the Cure: A History of Medicine in America (p. 39-40). Scribner. Kindle Edition.

13   Bliss, Michael. William Osler: A Life in Medicine. Kindle Locations 3309-3315 to 3316-3319. Kindle Edition.

14   Hopkins History

15   Moffit, R., 2011. Reforming Health Care on the Foundation of First Principles, 4999(1183).

16   Benjamin Rush in the Pennsylvania Ratification Convention, 12 December 1787 in http://csac.history.wisc.edu/pa_7.pdf

CHAPTER THREE:

EXCEPTIONALISM IN AMERICAN BIOETHICS

"Of all the dispositions and habits which lead to political prosperity, religion and morality are indispensable supports.... And let us with caution indulge the supposition that morality can be maintained without religion."

—George Washington, Farewell Address published on September 19, 1796.

The roots of American medical exceptionalism are to be found within our first principles that are derived from our secular government along with a society based on religious values, a combination that is unique in history, according to the conservative commentator on politics and religion, Dennis Prager.[1] According to Prager, and physician, Ronald Cherry,[2] our secular state was created when "Our Founding Fathers separated church from state, but they wisely did not separate God from state." While our Founding Fathers acknowledged God as the source of the Bibles, they expressly acknowledged Biblical morality as being foundational to our country, but not so the Church.

America is also unique in calling itself 'Judeo-Christian,' meaning that it recognizes the religions of the Old Testament, the Hebrew Bible, as well as the New Testament.[3] The author of the Declaration of Independence, Thomas Jefferson, explicitly uses precepts of both Bibles[3] in penning the chief source of our first principles, as does its physician signatory, Dr. Benjamin Rush.[4] And, President George Washington points out the importance to the nation of the link between religion and morality by saying in his Farewell Address that "the nation's morality cannot be maintained without religion."[5] And, he further reminds us that the Founding Fathers believed in the religious principles that "promote the protection of property, reputation, and life."[6]

While these great men acknowledged God as the source of both Bibles, and acknowledged Biblical values as being foundational to our country, they prohibited the establishment of a state Church. (First Amendment)[7] Biblical values are written directly into our founding documents and laws, with the express goal of preventing future totalitarian or tyrannical rule in America. It is because of our adoption of Biblical values, not the religions themselves, that we condemn the ACA as immoral. And, it is this "combination of keeping Judeo-Christian religious morality in the state, as opposed to the church, itself; and... setting up our laws based on reason and common sense [that]has contributed to the American Character, and to what is known as "American Exceptionalism."

Just as values derived from the Hebrew and Christian bibles have played foundational roles in American history, so too, do Judeo-Christian values figure heavily in the ethics of American healthcare. Up to the time of the Hopkins experience, professional behavior was primarily guided by the individual's core morality, beliefs in what was the right versus wrong medical actions to take in their medical practice. In time, an entirely new branch of medical ethics would arise. The new discipline, termed 'Bioethics' became the study of "ethical and moral implications associated with new biological discoveries and biomedical achievements, such as discovery of new drugs, innovation of medical devices and other bio-medical technologies including the game changing genetic engineering."[8] Each new achievement was accompanied by a constellation of ethical questions relating to the responsibilities of healthcare professionals in the context of biomedical innovations.

Passage of the ACA has placed questions of bioethics squarely in the public discourse. As a result of our country's heritage of strict religious principles, many within our society have retained a close identification with Judeo-Christian values according to Prager and Cherry.[2] The Biblical values of right and wrong, truth, liberty and equality,[2] and that life itself is a gift from God, are integral to our culture as are our notion of the rejection of evil, and our beliefs in justice, the Ten Commandments and the Golden Rule. The Founding Fathers acknowledged God as the source of our rights in their writings of our founding documents and laws, while at the same time excluding the Church. Biblical morality, not the Church or religion, combined with our secular government comprise our first principles which must be reflected in healthcare reform.

A certain segment of the public, as they have in other industrialized countries, has become thoroughly secularized, transforming toward non-religious values and institutions.[9] This segment might be expected to opt for alternative, non-religiously oriented healthcare reform values in the ACA as promoted by the Progressives. If we are to retain the Judeo-Christian values embraced by a majority of the population, we must re-dedicate ourselves to the first principles as handed down by our Founding Fathers.

Exceptionalism in American healthcare ethics began when the world's first national code of professional ethics was created more than 150 years ago at the founding of the American Medical Association (1847). "At that time," according to Audrey Kao, MD, PhD in the AMA Journal of Ethics,[10] "the AMA's Code of Medical Ethics was considered comparable in its revolutionary stance to the Declaration of Independence"[11] resulting in a new, strengthened contract between healthcare providers and society. Up to that time, the physician's role was implicit, requiring physicians to intuit what was expected of them. Societal responsibilities remained murky. From that time forward, healthcare delivery would be organized around standards set forth in that contract:

"Society granted physicians status, respect, autonomy in practice, and financial rewards on the expectation that physicians would be competent, altruistic, moral, and would address the healthcare needs of individual patients and society" said Cruess and Cruess[12], also in the AMA Journal of Ethics. This arrangement, although subject to changes in American culture, remained the essence of the social contract with healthcare until 2010, with passage of the ACA. Bio-ethical issues, a major component of healthcare reform, rests with the reformers as to the set of values that best suits their philosophy, and upon which healthcare reform will be built. Clearly, the ACA as a statement of Progressivism has been chosen in order to repudiate American first principles in favor of collectivism. With its values of the group over the individual, government makes all the rules and then in a one size fits all.

COLLECTIVIST HEALTHCARE SYSTEMS ARE IMMORAL AND UNDER-PERFORM

Government-controlled healthcare systems, whether termed collectivist, nationalist, universal, or single-payer, repudiate our long accepted values, and are thus immoral within the context of America's first principles. In addition, when they are compared, head-to-head, with our healthcare system, as it existed prior to 2010, collectivist systems always under-perform.

The United States was "the first nation founded on the premise that men are by nature free, and therefore that the purpose of government is, and must be, only the protection of that natural freedom," writes political philosopher, Daren Jonescu.[11] When President Obama promises to transform our system, he means away from American individualism, and toward dependency on government, couching the change with words like "compassion," or "fairness."[13] And with the "Government On Track To Make Up 66% of Healthcare Spending," as the Forbes headline reads, [14] limited government becomes a thing of the past. The Declaration of Independence, and the U.S. Constitution both state that liberty is an unalienable right, which makes the individual the fundamental unit of moral concern, imparting to each, a right to think and act as he sees fit, and to disregard any pressures that might be placed on him for not serving some "greater good". "No one, including groups and governments, has a moral right to force him to act against his judgment." Only individuals can act on their own judgment, keep and use the product of their efforts, and still accept the moral responsibilities of their actions, the personal standards of right and wrong. Collectivism often substitutes bogus ethical claims such as 'the greater good of a group' over the moral responsibility of the individual, or attempts to coerce an unnatural result such as forced equality[15] Only through immoral coercion against the inviolability of the individual, can the unnatural tenets of collectivism even occur. Therefore the reason collectivism, or socialized medicine, cannot work is because they are immoral. [16]

Even as we watch the ACA transform government and healthcare, a typical, government-run healthcare model called the Veterans Health Administration, the very symbol of the government's "largest integrated health care system,"[17][18][19][20] has already proven that government-run healthcare just doesn't work.[17][18][19][20] Our government proudly makes claims about the quality of and access to the program: "By sharing services between medical centers, Healthcare Systems allow VHA to provide Veterans easier access to advanced medical care closer to their homes." Patient advocates are available to help resolve concerns, so they claim, "about any aspect of your health care experience."

Despite best intentions, it took a whistleblower in the summer of 2014 to break the much-publicized Veterans Affairs healthcare scandal that [17][18][19][20] resulted from an attempt to create a government-run healthcare monopoly. Headlines read, "At least 40 U.S. veterans died waiting for appointments at the Phoenix Veterans Affairs Health Care system." Extended delays for appointments were covered up when up to 1,600 veterans were placed on secret waiting lists while being forced to wait months to see a doctor which accounted for the deaths. [17] [18] [19] [20] Remove all competition, and healthcare "will operate with all the efficiency of the post office and all the charm and compassion of the IRS," as Thomas J. DiLorenzo of the Ludwig Mises institute puts it.[21]

The most glaring fact about the 2014 VHA scandal was that the Secretary of Veterans Affairs apparently had no clue about what was going on with the scandal. Neither did the President of the United States. What will this or any president really know about the medical care that the government provides when it controls all of it?" That is why we must now return medical care to the sole management of patients and their physicians.[22]

Excessive governmental control is a form of paternalism, lulling the people into a sense of dependence upon the state.[23] We were first warned of this potential by Alexis de Tocqueville who admonished us of this "soft despotism."[24] Patients are likewise at risk of being robbed of their autonomy and self-reliance, of losing their freedoms to determine their own healthcare, and are forced to submit to the only types of highly regulated services that are offered. And doctors lose their freedom to choose how to practice medicine. Dependency erodes and erases our Judeo-Christian founding principles in favor of statism, the belief that the state should be in control of all aspects of the society, economy, and governance.

Even in countries whose culture has been traditionally democratic, such as the U.K., under their National Healthcare System, factions have grown that push for greater collectivism. Collectivist healthcare systems under-perform when compared with those operating in the free market, as they have no incentive to improve, and therefore tend to degenerate. In fact, the NHS is undergoing privatization in an attempt to save it altogether. [25]

In Nationalized healthcare systems, in order to pay for so-called 'free medical care' (usually meaning no payment at the point of service), rationing of care is necessarily built-in.[26] Extremely long waiting periods are required for appointments with doctors (usually worse for appointments with specialists), even longer waits for high-tech diagnostic tests, and longer waiting still for treatments that must be scheduled. In addition, oppressive taxes are raised in order to pay for the collectivist healthcare.[27]

Patient satisfaction, one meaningful expression of health-care quality, shows U.S. citizens overwhelmingly in favor of their pre-ACA healthcare system, compared with German, Canadian, Australian, New Zealand, and British citizens who believe even more strongly that their collectivist systems needed "fundamental change" or "complete rebuilding." A significant list of healthcare metrics showing better outcomes from treatments of common diseases shows the U.S. System performing better. [28]

The type of threat being served-up to us by the ACA robs us of the freedoms of healthcare providers to innovate, and for consumers to choose. Collectivism is at the opposite pole from the type of medicine described by William Osler who recognized that "variability is the law of life and as no two faces are the same, so no two bodies are alike and no two individuals react alike and behave alike under the abnormal conditions we know as disease."[29] This insight should lead us toward 'personalized medicine' and away from collectivist notions. The goal of personalized medicine is to optimize medical care and outcomes by scientifically determining specific diagnoses and best treatments for each individual patient.

COLLECTIVISM AND THE NECESSARY RATIONING AND ALLOCATION OF SCARCE MEDICAL RESOURCES

Rationing of scarce medical resources is a serious, ethical dilemma in any healthcare system. For example, which patient should receive a life-saving organ transplant when only one organ is available, and multiple patients are on a waiting list for that organ. Alternatively, allocation of scarce resources applies to making decisions as to who receives life-saving medications that may be running low during epidemics.[30] Rationing and allocation also apply to non-emergency resources such as the budget. After making promises to create a healthcare system that is free to all of its citizens, governments universally cut services to pay for it, resulting in reduced services usually starting with controversial procedures before being extended to the infrequent, or procedures deemed distasteful, or anti-social, by the regime.[31][32]

In healthcare systems such as in the U.S. before 2010, the first principle of emphasizing each individual's right to their choice of healthcare was manifested by delivery of full resources to each patient wherever possible. However, need to make 'micro-allocation' decisions are at times required. The threat that the powerful elites in collectivist (totalitarian) states would commandeer resources for their own use can be confirmed in a pair of real-life cases that occurred in the U.S. late in the first decade of the 21st century.

Case One - A prolific Democratic fundraiser and friend of Speaker of the House, Nancy Pelosi, was diagnosed with a terminal case of bone cancer (multiple myeloma) at the Mayo Clinic. Doctors there, eager to please the man that had also given over $1 million to the Clinic, informed him that one drug seemed effective against his cancer during testing in the laboratory. The last chance to save his life with that drug, however, was thwarted by its being approved only for treatment of other, non-cancerous disorders. The only way the drug could be legally used in this case was to have the drug's manufacturer give permission under special "compassionate use" rules that protect the drug-maker from receiving a black mark in case of an adverse outcome.

No amount of pleading by the family could get the manufacturer to release the drug in this case. Somehow – and the family still isn't sure how - "Pelosi cajoled the FDA to find a legal justification that let Mayo administer the drug, even without the [man-ufacturer's] consent. [33] Unfortunately, the drug ultimately failed to save his life.

Case Two - A ten year old girl with end-stage cystic fibrosis, a potentially fatal disease of the lungs, was denied consideration for a lung transplant because under policy at that time, only patients 12 years old or over could be placed on the list for adult lungs, and pediatric lungs were available for transplant only extremely rarely. Doctors in this case were also pushing to have the policy waived in this case saying that the patient was large enough that they could perform a successful transplant with adult lungs.[34]

When HHS Secretary, Kathleen Sebelius was petitioned to al-low the transplant, she called for a review of transplant policies, but refused to intervene because of the complex factors that go into the transplant-list formula.

The story, fortunately, had a successful conclusion. After the family sued to have the "Under 12" policy reversed, a national out-pouring of approval for the little girl lead to a one-year change that makes children younger than 12 eligible for priority on adult lung transplant lists, and created a mechanism that would allow doc-tors to request exceptions for their pediatric patients.[35] Happily, six months following the surgery she is riding her bicycle and doing well at home. [36]

The first case illustrates how elites can cause things to happen for their friends in any healthcare system, suggesting that in a col-lectivist systems the potential for meddling would be great. The second case points out that no rule should be inviolable when it comes to the individual in allocation of scarce resources. The case of a young child is likely to be overlooked by fixed policies in a collectivist system.

THE DOCTOR-PATIENT RELATIONSHIP AND IMPLICATIONS FOR HEALTHCARE REFORM

Beginning with the Hippocratic Oath (5th century B.C.), a shift took place in the focus from class-based medical care to selfless service of individual patients. This Oath is still taken by physicians today, forever "unit[ing] morality and medical craft in a way that speaks across the millennia."[37]

Based upon effective communication between doctor and patient, the doctor-patient relationship is as important today as it has been throughout the history of medicine. The communication is central to building effective clinical relationships, and it so affects patient satisfaction or dissatisfaction within the healthcare system, that it has come to define the 'good' doctor.[38] The doctor-patient relationship is inherently challenging for most physicians to achieve. And, the autonomy that allows for self-determination and liberty central to the relationship is threatened by the ACA. Knowledge of intrusion by the Government is likely to interfere with doctors as they interact with patients as they gather information, develop, and maintain a therapeutic relationship, and communicate information back to the patient.All of these functions are essential in a robust doctor-patient relationship and the channels have to remain clear. If a patient does not trust a doctor, any undue anxiety may prevent the patient from fully hearing all of the information imparted by the doctor.

The relationship between a doctor and patient will determine how well information is exchanged, and therefore directly impacts the quality and completeness of their interactions. According to Jenifer Fong Ha in the Ochsner Journal[39] "Effective doctor-patient communication is a central clinical function in building a therapeutic doctor-patient relationship, which is the heart and art of medicine. This is important in the delivery of high-quality health care. Much patient dissatisfaction and many complaints are due to breakdown in the doctor-patient relationship" Problems with any of these areas will lead to patient dissatisfaction because they will not benefit fully from the doctor's knowledge and skills. A consistent level of dissatisfaction among patients can lead to physician burnout. And a solid doctor-patient relationship is an important determinant in patient compliance with treatment plans.

With a positive and clear channel of trust and communication, patients feel that they are heard and supported by their doctor, and will be more likely to have an honest discussion, which can contain essential elements that provide a more honest and frank exchange that enhances the probability of a more accurate diagnosis, and more effective treatment.[40]

Direct government intrusion into the doctor-patient relationship is already at work by denying doctors their First Amendment rights of free speech. For example, doctors in Florida stand to pay a $10,000 fine, or even lose their license if they discuss whether or if their patient has a gun in the house, [41] and in Pennsylvania, doctors are gagged from discussing the health implications of hydraulic fracturing, or "fracking," in the process of drilling for natural gases that may be taking place in their own neighborhood. [42]

And worse, the very autonomy promised to both doctors and patients by the right of Limited Government, is removed. According to John Hoff of the Heritage Foundation, "the new law gives the Administration extensive authority to achieve broadly outlined goals, allowing it to control every aspect of health care finance and delivery and to impose its view of how the health care system should operate. The structure of the healthcare system will be determined by one central authority, reducing flexibility and denying Americans the ability to make their own choices." [43]

REFERENCES:

1   http://dennisprager.com/what-does-judeo-christian-mean/

2   The Judeo-Christian Values of America, Cherry, americanthinker.com ·
     September 15, 2007 http://www.americanthinker.com/articles/2007/09/
     the_judeochristian_values_of_a.html#ixzz3QWJSfDjh

3   Prager explains, "First, Judeo-Christian America has differed from
     Christian countries in Europe in at least two important ways. One is that
     the Christians who founded America saw themselves as heirs to the Old
     Testament, the Hebrew Bible, as much as to the New. And even more im-
     portantly, they strongly identified with the Jews. http://dennisprager.com/
     what-does-judeo-christian-mean/. The second meaning of Judeo-Chris-
     tian is a belief in the biblical God of Israel, in His Ten Commandments
     and His biblical moral laws. It is a belief in universal, not relative, morali-
     ty. It is a belief that America must answer morally to this God, not to the
     mortal, usually venal, governments of the world."

4   http://en.wikipedia.org/wiki/Judeo-Christian and American Judeo-Chris-
     tian values and the Declaration of Independence, renewamerica.com · by
     John Locke · February 1, 2015)

5   http://en.wikipedia.org/wiki/George_Washington%27s_Farewell_Address

6   http://en.wikipedia.org/wiki/George_Washington%27s_Farewell_Ad-
     dress#Religion.2C_morality.2C_and_education

7   http://www.law.cornell.edu/constitution/first_amendment

8   http://en.wikipedia.org/wiki/Bioethics

9   Uhlmann, E.L., American Moral Exceptionalism., (2008), pp.1–44.

10   http://journalofethics.ama-assn.org/2001/11/fred4-0111.html Kao, 2001.

11   On Restoring American Individualism, Daren Jonescu, March 31, 2012
     http://www.americanthinker.com/articles/2012/03/on_restoring_ameri-
     can_individualism.htl

12   http://journalofethics.ama-assn.org/2005/04/oped1-0504.html

13   http://humanevents.com/2013/08/20/the-myth-of-liberal-compassion/

14   http://www.forbes.com/sites/chrisconover/2012/08/07/takeover-govern-
     ment-on-track-to-make-up-66-of-healthcare-spending-obamacare

15   http://www.afcm.org/healthcareprinciples.html

16   http://www.americanthinker.com/articles/2007/09/the_judeochristian_
      values_of_a.html

17   The Government Health-Care Model The Wall Street Journal by Kirth
      Gersen https://www.instapaper.com/read/505865350 and http://www.
      va.gov/health/aboutvha.asp

18   http://www.theamericanconservative.com/articles/memorial-day-night-
      mare/

19   http://www.politico.com/story/2014/05/veterans-administration-scan-
      dal-106982.html

20   "A fatal wait: Veterans languish and die on a VA hospital's secret list,"
      Scott Bronstein and Drew Griffin, CNN Investigations updated 9:19 PM
      EDT, Wed April 23, 2014, http://www.cnn.com/2014/04/23/health/veter-
      ans-dying-health-care-delays/

21   http://mises.org/library/socialized-healthcare-vs-laws-economics

22   Veteran's Health Care: Harbinger for the Rest of Us? - Capitalism Maga-
      zine, capitalismmagazine.com , Richard E. Ralston, September 8, 2014

23   (http://www.johnlocke.org/lockerroom/lockerroom.html?id=21768) .

24   http://www.heritage.org/research/reports/2009/09/soft-despotism-democ-
      racys-drift-what-tocqueville-teaches-today

25   (http://www.dailymail.co.uk/health/article-2918003/NHS-forced-abandon-free-
      healthcare-says-Britain-s-doctor-warns-service-needs-radical-change.html)

26   Goodman's book- Priceless

27   http://www.thedailybell.com/exclusive-interviews/35799/-Wile-John-
      Goodman-The-Destruction-of-US-Healthcare-and-How-to-Fight-Back/

28   The Grass Is Not Always Greener - Cato Institute http://www.cato.org/
      sites/cato.org/files/pubs/pdf/pa-613.pdf

29   The same citations as the opening Golden Thread citation Address to
      the New Haven Medical Association (6 January 1903), published as "On
      the Educational Value of the Medical Society" in Yale Medical Journal,
      Vol. IX, No. 10 (April 1903), p. 325

30   Rationing and Allocating Scarce Medical Resources, Coursera Online
      course (https://www.coursera.org/course/rationing) May 20 to July 7, 2013
      Instructors Ezekiel J. Emanuel, MD, PhD University of Pennsylvania

31   Health Insurance (Part I): The Socialist Nightmare by Russell L. Blay-

lock, MD, Exclusive for HaciendaPublishing.com Article Published Date: Wednesday, August 19, 2009 http://www.haciendapub.com/articles/national-health-insurance-part-i-socialist-nightmare-russell-l-blaylock-md Freedom of choice is invariably lost. Decision-making in collectivist healthcare system is based upon benefit to the group at the expense of individuals.

32   Rationing and Allocating Scarce Medical Resources, Coursera Online course https://www.coursera.org/course/rationing May 20 to July 7, 2013 Instructors Ezekiel J. Emanuel, MD, PhD University of Pennsylvania

33   Pelosi pulled strings to let dying Dallas lawyer Baron try experimental cancer drug dallasnews.com · by Todd J. Gillman · August 24, 2010 http://www.dallasnews.com/news/columnists/todd-j-gillman/20100815-Pelosi-pulled-strings-to-let-dying-7500.ece

34   Kathleen Sebelius won't intervene in girl's lung transplant case CBS News June 4, 2013 http://www.cbsnews.com/news/kathleen-sebelius-wont-intervene-in-girls-lung-transplant-case/

35   http://www.cnn.com/2013/06/12/health/pennsylvania-girl-transplant/

36   http://abcnews.go.com/Health/sarah-murnaghan-pedals-forward-lung-transplant/story?id=22915748

37   MacDougall, 2010, Pg 70-78

38   http://www.ncbi.nlm.nih.gov/pubmed/19584762

39   Ochsner J. 2010 Spring; 10(1): 38-43 in http://www.ncbi.nlm.nih.gov/pmc/articles/PMC3096184/

40   http://www.ncbi.nlm.nih.gov/pmc/articles/PMC1496871/?tool=pmcentrez&report=abstract.

41   http://jama.jamanetwork.com/article.aspx?articleid=1104313

42   http://www.projectcensored.org/22-pennsylvania-law-gags-doctors-protect-big-oils-proprietary-secrets/

43   (http://www.heritage.org/research/reports/2010/09/implementing-obamacare-a-new-exercise-in-old-fashioned-central-planning

CHAPTER FOUR:

THE GREATNESS OF AMERICAN MEDICINE IN THE 20TH CENTURY

American medical exceptionalism in the early decades of the 20th century led to the most impressive era of scientific achievement in history. Our superior medical delivery system, evolving out of the Hopkins experiment, enabled Americans to enjoy the highest standards of healthcare in the world. American medicine was sought after by people from around the globe, confident that the world's best specialists would be capable of accurately diagnosing and treating their conditions where others could not.

According to the health economist, Scott Atlas MD, PhD, availability of specialists "has become a cherished part of our medical delivery in America. More leaders in the field, and the doctors and medical scientists who actually devise and develop the most important innovations in medical care, are found in the United States than any country."[1] Since 1945, biomedical research has been viewed as the essential contributor to improving the health of individuals and populations in both the developed and developing worlds.[2] For example, the availability of state-of-the-art diagnostic imaging technologies, interpreted by the best-trained radiologists, resulted in the most accurate diagnosis of diseases in the world[3]

Moreover, with the advent of clinician-scientists, the United States began conducting more clinical trials of new drugs on a variety of specific diseases than any country in the world. There is little doubt that the exceptional American medical model of healthcare remained intact throughout the 20th century and must serve as the model for healthcare reform.

THE EXISTING ETHICAL MILIEU

The American doctor's adherence to a code of ethics that includes the doctor-patient relationship remained the cornerstone of our healthcare system. In mid-twentieth century, an entirely new sub-set of medical ethics, 'bioethics,' emerged. Bioethics arose in response to new medical, ethical problems associated with the rapid advances in bio-medical technology. Bio-medical innovations began to drive the practice of medicine. Now, beyond the moral issues of doctors relating to patients, there were new drugs, dialysis machines, organ transplantation, cardio-respiratory resuscitation and support devices, electronically wired ICUs, as well as advanced surgical equipment and techniques, each one bearing the promise of greater longevity, reduction of the anxiety that accompanies the diagnosis of horrid diseases, and the easing of pain.[4]

Our healthcare system prior to the ACA was organized around the first principles of individuality and liberty. Our American ideals emphasize that each individual deserves the best care regardless of whether he/she is suffering from common ailments, or rare. Sustained, aggressive investment in research, and the promise of advancements in biomedical technology of the American ethos, began being shortchanged by the ACA.

THE ROLE OF PHYSICIAN SPECIALISTS IN 20TH CENTURY AMERICAN MEDICINE

So, how and why do the supporters of the ACA want to tear down the very system that has made our system exceptional? Let's first look at the essential role specialists have played in American medicine. According to economist and physician Scott Atlas, studies have clearly shown that specialty medical care not only results in superior outcomes to treatments that "extend the length and greatly improve the quality of life," but also results in cost savings."[1] In reality, it is early diagnosis and treatment by specialists that results in the highest quality healthcare at the lowest cost. The ACA is destroying one of the greatest assets of American healthcare -- specialty medicine.[1] In fact, it is the combination of advancements in biomedical technology along with specialty care that is the hallmark of American Medical exceptionalism.

To keep pace with growing medical knowledge, specialization has become increasingly complex, and specialty training more essential, not less, as the ACA would have it. This combination of science and training has helped to turn the tide in the epidemic of heart disease, stroke, and HIV/AIDS. Today people who suffer from these conditions are living longer and healthier than they did mere decades ago.

We also face a crisis as larger segments of the population of Americans enter seniority. Before the ACA, we were well on the way to positively redefining what it means to grow old. However, by cutting our force of specialists the whole idea of healthy aging will have to be reconsidered.[1] To care for the aging baby boomers the need for specialists will increase in order to take care of those with chronic conditions such as heart disease, cancer, stroke, diabetes, arthritis, COPD (Chronic Obstructive Pulmonary Diseases) and Alzheimer's disease. The Association of American Medical Colleges already estimates a deficit of 64,800 medical specialists by 2025. Further, the focus of the ACA on primary care will only increase the existing shortage of primary-care doctors by more than 65,000.

Despite the success of specialty medicine, the Medicare Independent Payment Advisory Board, (IPAB) a controversial 17-member appointed agency created in its current form by the ACA, has already recommended cuts to reimbursements for specialist doctors amounting to 16.7 percent over three years, followed by a freeze in spending equal to a 50 percent decrease in money for specialized care over the next 10 years. The ACA, by shifting "resources and prioritization to general care physicians at the expense of specialist care," intends to lower costs by making primary care physicians gatekeepers to specialists just as they were with Health Maintenance Organizations (HMOs) in the 1990's which advocated reductions in utilization as a major strategy to lower costs. The new iteration of IPAB with its near-autocratic decision making capabilities, and its mere presence threatens continued cuts to Medicare.[16]

The plan within the ACA to enhance the numbers of and emphasis on primary care physicians could have been helpful, per se. Primary care physicians include family practice specialists, internal medicine physicians who elect to act as primary care providers, pediatricians who fulfill that role for children, as well as general physicians who have licenses to practice after graduating from medical school and fulfilling a 1-2 year internship. However, it is not helpful to set up a primary care versus specialist mentality as is being done within the ACA. Primary care doctors practice most efficiently when they follow families and individuals over time, managing their health and well-being, and perform a monitoring function for the presence of serious impending disorders. Rather than acting as overly strict gatekeepers, when primary care physicians recognize early signs of serious diseases, timely referrals to the correct specialists is in their patients' best interest, as well as the financial well-being of the healthcare system.

Although skimping on diagnostic tests may reduce expenses initially, costs will increase dramatically as diagnoses are missed or delayed, thus delaying needed care. Diagnostic errors, which cause delayed treatment are the most costly and dangerous medical mistakes.[5] Americans demand more great medicine, not less, as is currently written into the ACA.

"Changing from a system of specialization to one dominated by primary care might be the most misguided part of the entire bill, and highly immoral as well."[1]

The ACA also stifles innovation in medical technology with punitive taxes and restricted access to important specialty care interventions and services. This move has economic consequences as well as medical ones. The ACA's medical device excise tax − on revenues, not just profits − is already destroying high-paying jobs for Americans and moving them overseas. By some estimates, the ACA will cause a loss of 45,000 jobs in the U.S.

Further cuts in technology-based specialty procedures have already been proposed by IPAB, with its unprecedented power to reduce Medicare payments. The Secretary of HHS is required to implement these cuts, and neither Congress nor the courts can overturn them. Although language in the law prohibits overt rationing of care, rationing will be the result.

Even Howard Dean, Democratic former Governor of Vermont and Chair of the Democratic National Committee recently warned, "The IPAB is essentially a healthcare rationing body. By setting doctor reimbursement rates for Medicare and determining which procedures and drugs will be covered and at what price, the IPAB will be able to stop certain treatments its members do not favor by simply setting rates to levels where no doctor or hospital will perform them."[6]

The access to primary care should be increased and made more affordable by expanding outpatient clinics in retail settings and allowing certain routine services to be delivered by well-trained allied healthcare providers such as nurse practitioners and physician assistants. We must look to the future for a new paradigm where we promote and leverage a trained work force, along with technological advances, to participate in the formidable tasks ahead. Those tasks include managing the growth in numbers of patients who will gain access to the healthcare system such as the previously uninsured, as well as the growing number of seniors and others with chronic illnesses that require ongoing management where previously, many of those diseases proved fatal.

AMERICAN MEDICINE AND THE REVOLUTION IN SCIENTIFIC AND MEDICAL TECHNOLOGY

Part of the success of U.S. healthcare delivery resulted from state-of-the-art diagnostic imaging devices that were made widely available to consumers. In turn, they could benefit through the cost savings enjoyed by having nearby diagnostic facilities, with low waiting times, and expert specialists in radiology, either present on campus, or through online connections (tele-radiology) to interpret the studies, and recommend next-steps to treating specialists.

Prior to the ACA, entrepreneurs were able to purchase these devices and share in the profits that they generated. Specialists, such as radiologists who interpret diagnostic images, also invested in the CT and MRI scanners. Although it was highly regulated by the government, entrepreneurs and physicians, the so-called supply-side of the equation, was allowed to take advantage of America's first principles, use the (partially) free market and competition to drive down fees, and provide incentives for industry to develop newer and better devices. Such strategies in the future by providers (the supply side), will be key to lowing prices through competition and innovation.[7]

IS THE COST OF TECHNOLOGY WORTH IT?

"The value of technological advances in medicine has not been lost on the American public. In studies, 80 percent of Americans say that being able to get the most advanced tests, drugs, medical procedures and equipment is 'very important' or 'absolutely essential'; a full 67 percent say that technologies such as digital imaging and advances in health information technology will improve patient care and or reduce medical costs, while only 10 percent think these advances cost more than they are worth." [1]

Although it is widely accepted that technological changes have accounted for the bulk of medical care cost increases over time, those costs may well be viewed as acceptable in a country that so highly values the "pursuit of happiness". The economist, David Cutler proposes that in order to fully understand the importance of technology in healthcare, it must be measured by its effect on specific diseases rather than its across the board impact as previously reported.

The ACA threatens to reduce one of medicine's main missions to subsidize the biomedical research.[8] Rather than cutting funding for technological research and development across the board, it makes sense to take into account technological cost-effectiveness in specific diseases. In a landmark scientific paper,[9] Cutler studied cost-effectiveness of technology in the treatment of five specific disorders: heart attacks, low birth-weight in infants, depression, cataracts, and breast cancer. By then calculating monetary values attributed to technology for increased longevity, improved quality of life, and increased productivity (spending less time away from work), he determined that the estimated monetary benefit of technological change is much greater than the costs in all of the disorders except for breast cancer where the costs and benefits were about of equal magnitude.[9]

Unless we do something to change what is already written in the ACA, funding of future breakthroughs in technology will be threatened. ACA decision-makers believed that the high costs of technology in medicine should be arbitrarily reduced in order to contain costs. This conflicts with America's first principles that promote such values as aggressive biomedical research and development in pursuit of longer, and improved quality of life. Cutler's technique makes it possible to guide future decision-makers on a disease-by-disease basis.

A TRIUMPH OF THE HEART-PREVENTION

One dramatic example of Cutler's work is his analysis of medical technology in the diagnosis and treatment of cardiovascular (heart and blood vessel) disease. Between 1950 and 1990, the mortality rate for sufferers of cardiovascular disease fell by 60 percent, and it continues to fall to this day, while survivors realize improvements in their quality of life. [10] However, the cost of achieving that improvement has been estimated at over $110 billion annually in the U.S. "To determine whether this expenditure was worth it, the authors consider what they call the admittedly controversial index of the dollar value of a year of life. They conclude that we are better off having spent our money on heart attack care than we would have been if the money had been spent elsewhere. Moreover, in view of the value of the resulting improved health, the implication is that the cost of living for heart attack victims is actually falling." [10]

However, the value of Cutler's work does not stop there.[9] Appreciating that in the specific instance of cardiovascular disease, spending in biomedical research is so potentially great from a monetary return on investment, further aggressive, follow-on research is warranted. Such research has the potential to reveal new, game-changing approaches to disease management. For example, further research in computerized imaging demonstrated how screening with the CT and MRI scanners have revealed ultra-early lesions that can be prevented from ever becoming a threat to the patient's life.

The innovation in the CT scanner that enabled this change was made possible only through continued research and development. This work led to the ability to take faster and faster scans. Being ever in motion through beating, the heart, and heart vessels could not be accurately imaged by the slower CT scanners. However, when the rate of taking images rose to match the rate of the beating heart, CT images could be performed that reveal the details of the arteries, allowing diagnoses of any obstruction within their central canals.

The success of CT scanning led to further research that yielded new, high-speed CT scanners with the capability to determine the presence of atherosclerosis (blockage due to fatty deposits) inside arteries non-invasively. Now symptomatic patients could be diagnosed earlier and more safely, enabling timely treatment by the least invasive modalities—such as angioplasty balloons—or, aggressive surgery when deemed necessary by the scanner.

Non-invasive computerized imaging to screen for early signs of disease has opened up an approach to diagnosis that could eliminate most heart attacks or strokes. Routinely scheduled screening at various ages, before symptoms occur, could pick up evolving problems years earlier when it is still possible to treat them with less-aggressive modalities such as medication and lifestyle change. This same strategy could also be utilized in pre-screening of cancer, when silent tumors may only be a few cells in size. Only continued funding for biomedical research will enable this potential to become cost-effective.

WILL WE ALLOW TECHNOLOGY TO TRIUMPH?

It is estimated that 80 percent of all the innovation in healthcare comes from the U.S. healthcare system. American companies dominate the $350 billion global medical device industry, with 32 of the 46 medical technology companies, each with more than $1 billion in annual revenue. Research in drug discovery and biomedical technology is dominated by the U.S. And, according to the Secretary of the Department of Health and Human Services, "advances in medical technology continue to transform the provision of health care while they lengthen and improve quality of life." It is difficult to argue with the CDC statement that, "It is almost inconceivable to think about providing healthcare in today's world without medical devices, machinery, tests, computers, prosthetics, or drugs." [11]

Yet the ACA goes a long way to reduce efforts of continued medical innovations. Even with the profitability and potential growth of the industry, innovation investments have become a fertile area for cutting costs according to ACA decision makers who seek to reduce costs by cutting funding for research and development in biomedical technology. Even careful policies that attempt to cut funding without interfering in advancement, do just that. Less than aggressive attitudes toward research have been shown to retard progress. [9] This is a powerful argument against being reliant on the government to make all investment decisions, which in the case of the ACA, wrong-headedly seeks to engineer equality through a lowest common denominator approach rather than allowing entrepreneurs to drive innovation development.

Innovation is further hurt by taxation on medical devices. The 2.3 percent ACA medical device tax on sales of medical devices will hurt innovation and small businesses through the impact on research and development, as well as employment in the industry. The tax has already resulted in employment reductions of approximately 14,000 workers. [12] Prices on items such as stents and artificial joints, used more often as a consequence of aging, will go up as higher manufacturing costs are passed on to consumers, causing seniors to suffer disproportionately. [13]

By curtailing medical innovation and economic growth, the tax will make more expensive exactly the kind of innovative, cost-saving health care that experts recognize as the most beneficial in the U.S. health care system. [14] Also to be considered are chronic illnesses, perhaps the greatest challenge to rising costs of healthcare. They are often manageable but incurable, and account for more than 75% of healthcare spending. [15]

Although chronic diseases are more common among older adults, they affect people of all ages and are now recognized as a leading health concern of the nation. Growing evidence indicates that a comprehensive approach to prevention can save tremendous costs and needless suffering.[11] A warning such as that should incentivize innovative entrepreneurs who offer the greatest chance to tackle the challenge by creating opportunities for technological progress, not barriers.

MY PERSONAL IMAGING REVOLUTION

Nothing is more compelling, in most instances, than first-hand experience to shed light on the significance of revolutionary breakthroughs in medical science. My experience in the imaging revolution came about thanks to the invention of the CT scanner, or Computerized Axial Tomogram (CAT).

REVOLUTION IN THE AIR

Looking east from Shockoe Hill in Richmond, the site of the Medical College of Virginia (MCV), you can follow Broad Street as it winds up Church Hill toward Old St. John's Episcopal, just a few blocks away. Its' tall spire becomes visible with the sunrise. However, no spire had yet been erected on the small single-story frame church on March 23, 1775. The Second Virginia Convention met there that night, instead of at the Raleigh Tavern down the road in Williamsburg. They met to debate encroachment of civil rights by the British Monarchy. Soon, they were to become witnesses to the kindling of the Torch of Liberty. Richard Henry Lee, Thomas Jefferson, and George Washington sat transfixed when another delegate rose, and delivered the most powerful speech ever given:

"Gentlemen may cry peace, peace—but there is no peace. Forbid it, Almighty God! I know not what course others may take; but as for me, give me liberty, or give me death!"

—PATRICK HENRY
THE OLD ST. JOHN'S EPISCOPAL CHURCH, RICHMOND, VIRGINIA, MARCH, 1775

Standing on Shockoe Hill some mornings, you become transfixed by the sounds of revolution in the air, and feel the crushing impact, as if it was yesterday instead of yesteryear. MCV is indeed situated in the midst of history that bore witness to a birth of a Nation, as well as to the worst man-made disaster to take place within our shores, the carnage of the Civil War. Look to the left and let your imagination bring to life the Civil War era Chimborazo Hospital, the largest hospital that ever existed in the western world, sitting on the bluff less than a mile due west. It was said to have had as many as 7000 beds with one of the lowest mortality rates of any hospital in the Civil War. Between 1861 and 1865, Chimborazo Hospital treated approximately 75,000 patients, more than any other facility in either the North or South.

However, another revolution was taking place in 1976 with the introduction of the CT scanner to brain surgery. Few medical innovations have had the overnight impact on the course of medicine than did the CT scanner upon neurosurgery, which radically, though positively, altered almost its entire diagnostic and operative procedure manuals when the first of the scanners' primitive images began coming through. Their impact on me, a first-year neurosurgery resident, in the Emergency Room, struggling to diagnose the causes of comas in patients with head trauma from high-speed motor vehicle accidents, was like that of a doctor in the trenches when the first of Fleming's new penicillin arrived. Neurosurgeons, in particular, have been in a protracted war against the ravages of motor-vehicle accidents. Over 53,000 people would die from traumatic brain injuries due to motor vehicle accidents that year. However, many thousands of other accident victims would survive long enough to make it to the Emergency Room, where rapid decisions by the neurological trauma team would determine life, death and the quality of one's functions. That was the front line for me, where I lived, grappling with one of the toughest problems in all of medicine.

The most serious immediate problem to solve when patients

arrive in the ER in acute coma following serious brain trauma is to determine whether the coma was caused by the direct injury to brain cells at the time of the accident, or whether it is due to a complication that develops after the injury, such as a clot of blood pressing on the brain. But how can you tell? You cannot look through the skull. At least you could not before the CT.

In order to determine if comatose patients had "surgically treatable" blood clots prior to the advent of the CT scanner, the neurosurgery resident (there was no time to wait for a professor to come in from home in the middle of the night) would perform a surgical procedure in the Emergency Room to instill air into the mid-line ventricles of the brain. The shadow of that small amount of air on a skull x-ray might yield indirect evidence as to the possible cause of the coma.

My small part in the computerized imaging revolution began when Sir Godfrey Hounsfield, an English electrical engineer who, with funding obtained directly through sales of Beatles albums, developed the diagnostic technique of x-ray computed tomography. This technique not only safely opened "a virtual window on the brain," but gave us, non-invasive, three-dimensional pictures of the brain inside the skull. Within minutes (now seconds), the cause, and appropriate treatment could be determined by reviewing three-dimensional images projected on a screen.

As I would come to understand later that first night when I had a moment to reflect, everything was different now. Whether today or tomorrow, all structural diseases of the brain and spinal cord would be diagnosable for free—free from complications. Moreover, if one could peer through the thick bone of the skull or spine, would the revolution not extend to cover all other organs of the body? I now often reflect on my luck in being able to experience neurosurgery before-and-after the advent of computer generated images. That has a lot to do with why I am writing this book. I can still look out from Shockoe Hill and give a shout-out toward Old St. John's Episcopal, to thank some of the men who made this possible.

REFERENCES:

1   Scott Atlas Book, Excellence, 2012.

2   Moses et al, 2011, Pgs. 567-571.

3   Kangarloo, H., Improving diagnosis through teleradiology.

4   http://www.ncbi.nlm.nih.gov/pmc/articles/PMC1447035 /

5   http://qualitysafety.bmj.com/content/early/2013/03/27/bmjqs-2012-001550.
    abstract

6   The Affordable Care Act's Rate-Setting Won't Work, Experience tells
    me the Independent Payment Advisory Board will fail. The Wall Street
    Journal Online HOWARD DEAN, July 28, 2013, http://online.wsj.com/
    news/articles/SB10001424127887324110404578628542498014414

7   Goodman Book- Priceless

8   http://www.chicagotribune.com/news/ct-aca-research-sidebar-met-
    20140811-story.html

9   David M. Cutler and Mark McClellan Is Technological Change In Medi-
    cine Worth It? Health Affairs , 20, no.5 (2001):11-29

10 http://www.nber.org/digest/oct98/w6514.html

11 http://www.cdc.gov/chronicdisease/resources/publications/aag/chronic.
    htm

12   http://advamed.org/res.download/417

13 http://www.forbes.com/sites/theapothecary/2013/09/14/obamacares-medi-
    cal-device-excise-tax-early-evidence-suggests-significant-harm/

14 http://thehill.com/blogs/congress-blog/economy-bud-
    get/194534-kill-the-medical-device-tax#ixzz3B82ilyan

15 http://www.fightchronicdisease.org/sites/fightchronicdisease.org/files/
    docs/GrowingCrisisofChronicDiseaseintheUSfactsheet_81009.pdf

16 (Obamacare's Supporters Are Living In The Past, Which Is Where
    Healthcare Quality Will Remain, Scott Atlas, forbes.com · September 22,
    2013 http://www.forbes.com/sites/scottatlas/2013/09/22/obamacares-sup-
    porters-are-living-in-the-past-which-is-where-healthcare-quality-will-re-
    main/

CHAPTER FIVE:

AMERICAN MEDICINE IN THE AGE OF GLOBALISM

OUR INCOMPARABLE SYSTEM

American medical delivery before 2010 was clearly the best in the world based upon a wide array of important benchmarks. Outcomes from treatment of the most serious diseases soared. Specialist physicians in all areas of medical practice, as well as state-of-the art diagnostic and therapeutic technologies were conveniently available locally in most communities. Together with adequate numbers of primary care physicians, waiting times were the lowest of any country—hours or days instead of weeks or months. These services were available to all Americans, as well as to a multitude of people who chose to travel from around the globe, including heads of State.

The U.S. healthcare system was also considered, by many, as the best in ways not routinely thought about in head-to-head comparisons with other countries. U.S. healthcare had been a pioneer in the world in providing services specifically aimed at assuring the quality and qualifications of professionals and facilities so that they were above reproach. In traveling to many countries, learning about different healthcare systems, I learned, sometimes at the behest of local and national governments, of the bogus credentialing of much of the professional work force. The United States has lead the way in preventing this from occurring in America for more than a century.

Physicians' Credentialing

Each country that I visited had serious problems in verifying the credentials of their professional staffs. In actuality, a large number of physicians had never attended medical school or residency training and were deceptively practicing with false credentials. Hospitals often had poor hygiene, and privacy of medical records was routinely breached. Standards in the U.S, by comparison, were incomparable: [1] All physicians had to possess current, verifiable licenses to practice medicine, issued by the state(s) (not federally) in which the practice, or, post-graduate training took place.

Accreditation of Medical Schools

Less than half of all countries with medical schools have any type of medical education accreditation, according to a 2008 study in the Journal of Medical Education. [2] Association of American Medical Colleges, began in 1876, when only 22 medical schools existed in the U.S. Since then that body has provided a standard for medical education for the over one-hundred sixty medical schools in the U. S. today.

Accreditation of Medical Specialists
(Board Certification),

The American Board of Medical Specialties (ABMS) exists to approve 24 different medical specialty boards in the development and use of standards in the ongoing evaluation and certification of physicians. The ABMS, formed in 1933, is recognized as issuing

Board Certification, the "gold standard" in physician qualification. There are other new Specialty Accreditation entities around the world that have much lower, less rigorous standards. [3]

Accreditation of Hospitals

Traditionally (up to the 1960's) in the U.S., the health care system relied on credentialing mechanisms, such as licensure, registration, and certification by professional societies and specialty boards, to ensure the quality of clinical care. Beginning in the late 1950's, the Joint Commission on Accreditation of Hospitals[4] an independent, not-for-profit organization, began certifying hospitals and continued until covering more than 20,500 healthcare organizations and programs in the United States. The Joint Commission on accreditation and certification, formed many years before any other country, is recognized nationwide as a symbol of quality that reflects an organization's commitment to meeting required performance standards.

The Public Health Service

The Public Health Service is a government agency within the U.S. Department of Health and Human Services, which came into being in 1798. The term "public health" connotes savings of lives on a community-wide scale. Untold people have been spared pain, misery, and death from such things as transmission of communicable diseases, unsanitary environments, and unsafe food and water.

Medical Malpractice Insurance

The U.S. has had a system for compensating patients for professional wrongdoing through medical malpractice (professional liability) insurance, which has been present in some form since the 1840's. The ethical environment in the U.S. has provided this form of redressing aggrieved patients and families well before any other country. Many still lack these services today.

Peer Review

Processes, including one that was developed by William Osler, Peer Review Conferences, are conducted within teaching institutions in order to evaluate the work of individual residents in training by one's colleagues. Regular conferences to examine and constructively correct potential clinical medical mistakes made by residents in training, has become important in the quality assurance process in U.S. healthcare. Peer review is also an integral part of verifying truth and accuracy in determining an academic paper's suitability for publication.

Health Insurance

The U.S. Healthcare system included health insurance earlier and with wider coverage than any other country in the world. Health insurance became widely available in 1929, with private hospitalization insurance to assure hospitals were paid for delivered services. In 1939, private insurance to pay physicians for delivered services for office visits, house calls, and doctor services in the hospital was made available, and with World War II, employer-based health insurance began.

THE WHO HYSTERIA:
1. THE WORLD REPORT OF 2000—THE BELL WAS RUNG

Despite its excellence as steadily documented in the world's medical and scientific literature, American healthcare was to endure a barrage of criticisms and distortions about its quality and costs, beginning in 1960, and escalating steadily up to the passage of the ACA in 2010. This campaign of unwarranted criticism and misinformation was carried out in order to further the goals of a group of foreign and domestic parties with a poorly hidden collectivist agenda. It aimed at demoralizing the people of America into being ashamed of their healthcare system, even though a majority had repeatedly continued to respond to surveys that showed their satisfaction with their own healthcare. The campaign was aimed at dissuading world leaders and healthcare decision makers of the exceptionalism of U.S. healthcare.

Americans understood, from personal experience, that American medical care was outstanding. Americans also understood what they could lose in a centralized, government-controlled healthcare system in which government is empowered to exercise control over the most personal decisions. It was precisely such knowledge that represented a threat by those with Progressive political motivation that sought to force U.S. healthcare off of its moral moorings. [5]

Through a willful, persistent campaign to besmirch the quality of U.S. healthcare, and in a campaign to fuel the aspirations of domestic and global collectivists, a bell was rung by economists, government officials, insurers, and academics who shared a worldview that ran counter to America's values,. This bell of propaganda reverberated, advocating greater government involvement in healthcare, implementation of a single-payer system of healthcare delivery in the U.S. and a rejection of America's first principles. Sadly, the bell could not be 'unrung.' Why was this campaign undertaken, by whom, how accurate were the criticisms compared to the true nature of U.S. healthcare? [6] And most importantly, how damaging was this campaign?

2. THE REPORT

In 2000, the World Health Organization (WHO, Geneva) published a report, "The World Health Report 2000 - Health systems: improving performance," dubbed by Hoover Institution Senior Fellow, Scott Atlas, MD PhD, as the "Worst Study Ever?" [7] for its bias, and total lack of scientific validity.

The putative reason behind the study was to compare health systems in its 191 member states, in order to look for quantifiable differences related to health system performance that would help "strengthen the scientific foundations of health policy." [6]

The "Report" was to become the first of its kind to publish a ranking of all 191 countries based upon the performance of their healthcare system. The report [8] ranked the U.S. healthcare system as 37th in the world in overall performance behind such countries as those with Nationalized Healthcare systems (Canada, the UK and Germany), but also risibly behind the likes of Morocco, Greece, Andorra, and the Sultanate of Oman. [9] The study proved fraudulent, and a classic example of disinformation. The report became a vehicle used to spread deceptive statements in order to achieve its' creators' hidden objectives.[10]

Over the years, in fact, several world-class scientists have come forward to thoroughly discredit the method by which the WHO report was performed, and to point out the bias behind the uneven weight given to countries based-upon their progressiveness. [11]

There are those in the United States and elsewhere in the world who maintain an unswerving derision of America and American medicine, precisely because of the propaganda campaign that began with the World Health Organization (WHO) report in 2000. [9] The hysteria that was provoked, primarily by America's ranking of #37, set the "Report's" perverted narrative in motion, as if it figured in a game of Chinese Whispers. The findings of the WHO Report were passed, verbatim, from article to article for over a decade. The meme spread throughout professional journals, and popular articles forming a deliberate, false narrative about U.S. healthcare.

3. THE EDITOR-IN-CHIEF COMES FORWARD

In this curious case, we have been handed a smoking gun by none other than the Editor-in-Chief of the WHO 2000 Report, himself, Philip Musgrove, PhD. Dr. Musgrove, for personal reasons, came forth and admitted to his own bad faith intentions in two

highly regarded medical journals, The Lancet, in 2003, and in fol-
low-up comments in the New England Journal of Medicine:

Dr. Philip Musgrove is quoted in the The Lancet[12] admitting to
the most grievous, but purposeful actions:

"The attainment values in WHO's World Health Report 2000
are spurious: only 39% are country-level observations. The responsiveness indicators are not comparable across countries; and three
values obtained from expert informants were discarded in favour of
imputed values. Indices of composite attainment and performance
are based on imputations and thus are also meaningless. Member
governments were not informed of the methods and sometimes
suffered unjust criticism because of the rankings. Judgments about
performance should be based on real data, represent methodologi-
cal consensus, be built from less aggregated levels, and be useful for
policy." [12]

Musgrove attempts to rationalize his bizarre and confusing behavior: "Fortunately...the report appears to make very little con-
nection between the results of the performance analysis and the
implications for undertaking functions [of health systems.]" [12]

Important associates and interested parties were unethically kept
in the dark about the findings until the eve of its publication when
they could not add any reactions or comments to the report: [12]

"Text authors were told essentially nothing about how some of the
indicators were estimated until near the end of the report's production."

"The result of this way of making the numbers was [sic] that
'Ministers of Health of the world may have felt, the day the report
was published, in the position of parents whose children had been
given grades in courses in which they did not know they were enrolled[12]. Several WHO representatives and liaison officers were also
taken by surprise. As some of them explained to me, the advance
copies of the report and press materials they were given could not
enable them to explain to outraged or baffled officials where the
numbers came from. Only 39% of the indicator values represent
real data, which falls to 18.5% if disability adjusted life expectancy

is set aside. This indicator was the only one not imputed by regression for 118 of the 191 member states of WHO."[12]

"Only 39% of the indicator values represent real data, which falls to 18.5% if disability adjusted life expectancy is set aside." [12]

Musgrove attempts to justify the report based upon intentions. His explanations appear as bizarre as his conclusions: "The supposition [was] that no-one [in the research community] was adequately concerned with [comparative] health-system problems, thus [sic] a ranking was needed to call attention to them." Also, "The assertion that nobody would have paid attention to an incomplete analysis restricted to real data [sic]. Possibly a more evidence-based analysis would have attracted less notice, because policy-makers pay too much attention to scorecards—partly because WHO and other organisations [sic] push them to do so." [12]

There have been other attempts to white-wash this report by referring to it as "courageous" in an attempt to stimulate needed research in the area of comparative health systems performance, and place it on the political agenda; and that its' faults were only "technical" in nature. [13]   Despite these attempts to justify the study, Martin McKee, a Professor of European Public Health at the London School of Hygiene and Tropical Medicine, said, "The World Health Survey promised to fill a major gap in our knowledge but it was effectively stillborn." [13]

The unusual admission by Chief Editor, Philip Musgrove, PhD. demonstrates how morally dispicable the report was, regardless of the motives. He has admitted to falsifying and fabricating data used throughout the report. Any notion that American healthcare exceptionalism should be tarnished by this report is unjust. The bell must be unrung.

4. THE DIRECT IMPACT

An admission coming years after the release of the report, even by its' Editor-in-Chief, had no mitigating consequences on the effects of the successful fraud. The dramatic headline that the "United States healthcare system ranks 37th in the world" has been allowed to propagate, unfettered, to the point that it has become a meme on the Internet. It has become, perhaps, the most damaging scientific hoax of the 20th century. It alone has been largely responsible for manipulating public attitudes toward U.S. Healthcare. The report "Provided supporters of President Barack Obama's transformative healthcare legislation with a data-driven argument for swift and drastic reform."[5] In October 2008, according to Scott Atlas, candidate Obama used the study to claim, "29 other countries have a higher life expectancy and 38 other nations have lower infant mortality rates" both of which are factually untrue.[5]

Largely as a result of the report's impact, a consistent, popular belief that collectivist, Universal Healthcare systems are clinically and socio-economically preferable to that of the U.S. system, remains intact. There is no doubt that this was the sought-after conclusion of its authors. However, the conclusion is factually incorrect. Deception through disinformation is a hallmark of the statists, because the truth alone is not persuasive to most people. Further, this case shines a light on the hidden agenda of the WHO, and demonstrates to the world the tactics employed by global activists, and goes to the proof that Universal Healthcare systems cannot stand alone on their merits.

It is of paramount importance to understand the fraudulent nature of this report since it has become the central, albeit, factually incorrect nucleus of the popular criticism of American healthcare, resulting in the singular, incessantly repeated narrative: "The world's richest country spends more of its money on healthcare while getting less in return than almost every other nation." It has been used to ridicule the U.S. and its' healthcare system, in order to make both vulnerable as targets for takeover and radical reform.

PROOF OF THE WHO'S INTENT TO DAMAGE THE U.S.

"The World Health Organization took great pains not to announce publicly that the U.S. Healthcare system actually ranked first in the world in terms of responsiveness to patients' needs for choice of provider, dignity, autonomy, timely care, and confidentiality. In other words, "where it matters most to patients, the U.S. system excelled." This would suggest that its "public chastisement has little to do with America's quality and delivery of healthcare services." [14]

5. THE WHO'S HIDDEN AGENDA

The World Health Organization, prior to passage of the ACA, primarily faulted the United States for its failure to impose mandatory insurance (Universal), and not offering its' version of social welfare programs (welfare state) to all of its citizens--in other words, for being a free country with independent citizens. The report putatively measured indices of "quality," while unknown to its' readers, ranking of member healthcare systems was based solely on a measure of whether the country's healthcare system was or was not on a course to adopt Universal care, the goal of socialists (statists). [14]The report's authors and so-called investigators self-determined, without regard to any semblance of scientific data, which member country would be ranked above others based upon the WHO's own priorities regarding the allocation of national resources. By surreptitiously changing the conventional indices of "quality," the authors manufactured results without announcing this change ahead of release of the study. [14]

The WHO, an agency of the United Nations (UN), "has been surrounded by an aura of humanism and social concern that has protected it from close scrutiny." [15] However, both organizations are "heavily involved in propaganda in the guise of apolitical neutrality." WHO policies have been demonstrated to cause damage to developing countries with cultures that resemble ours in entrepreneurship, competition, and market values. [16]

I wrote "A Clean Bill of Health" in order to set the record straight, that the greatness of American medical care runs deep. Its origins are as impressive as that of our nation. The revolutionary Hopkins Experiment built exceptionalism into American medicine, and it has been enhanced and tested repeatedly for over a century. The 20th century brought unimagined achievements, innovations and a standard of care that could not be surpassed. However, the continued reverberation of the bell that could not be unrung, offered opportunists a false rhetoric based upon bad science with which to disparage American medicine in order to achieve their ends—their hidden collectivist agenda.[16] What are those ends?

6. THE HEALTHCARE AND THE MONEY TRAIL

In order to counter-balance the weightiness of the WHO report, it is essential to understand why it was so important, for those involved, to perpetrate this scheme. WHO's hidden collectivist agenda"* is now a matter of record.* Collectivist goals include a "New Universalism" and "New Global Health System"* (note: Health not 'Healthcare" system), a typical utopian dream that would surreptitiously rob the United States of its' treasure, to be redistributed freely among developing countries for purposes other than healthcare development. "It is entirely possible that improved health care may not be the primary goal of countries seeking the American dollar. The other 190 member countries of the World Health Organization may view dollars designated for healthcare as a meal ticket for purchases not directly related to medical services....And, given the opportunity, they would readily place control of every person's earnings and every patient's care into a few powerful hands." [14]

The United Nations' Universal Declaration of Human Rights claims that everyone has a right to healthcare. Of course, there's no such thing as free healthcare. The government has no money of its own which means that it cannot "give" anyone health care without first taking away something from someone else (i.e. taxpayers) [14] Such a claim represents the fundamental underlying motive in the campaign to disparage the U.S. healthcare system by global statists: Their hidden agenda to siphon monies off of American taxpayers in order to add to the wealth of those in power in other collectivist states.

Reaching out to other countries with aid might be a morally laudable goal of the American government. However, when the government undertakes such action, Americans have the right to know where their money is going and for what purpose. The right to choose how their property is being used is spelled out in America's first principles of being able to maintain the "fruits of their labor." Collectivists "dismiss the ethics inherent in earning, in order to keep, and control the fruits of others' labors." [17]

7. HEAD-TO-HEAD WITH OMAN

Little did I know, that when I visited a small country lying on the mouth of the Persian Gulf, one that I had scarcely heard of prior to my first trip to the region in 2002, that I would be thrust directly into the WHO ranking controversy. Of course, this coincidence affected my desire to chronicle my experiences someday. The visit would be the first of many to the region over the next eight years, and would form a counter-point to my working knowledge of the U.S. healthcare system.

The Sultanate of Oman is located on the southeast tip of the Arabian Peninsula, with a thousand mile coastline on the Indian Ocean extending from the entrance of the Strait of Hormuz into the Persian Gulf on the North, to its' border with the Republic of Yemen to the Southwest. Oman was to become an unlikely, albeit

lovely and exotic spot to serve as a defining rubric in my search
to answer a vexing healthcare puzzle, and to propel me into a decade long study of comparative healthcare systems of the world,
and ultimately, to write a book that I hoped might play a role in
restoring the great U.S. Healthcare system, and protecting it from
decimation.

I first traveled to Oman at the invitation of then U.N. Ambassador (Oman), H.E. Hunaina Sultan Ahmed Al Mughairy. I was
asked to consult on the benefits of telemedicine, tele-radiology,
and other online medical delivery products that I had been re-
searching along with a study group of well-regarded scientists and
entrepreneurs in California. I was also to tour the regional medical
facilities, led by one of the Royal Physicians. I was eager to compare my observations of the Omani "Healthcare Renaissance" with
the published findings by the WHO.

En route to the region, I read "The World Health Organization ("WHO") 2000 Report, Health Systems: Improving Performance," [18] that listed a ranking of its' 191 member states according
to a group of three measurements. Oman ranked first in one mea-
surement, healthcare systems' efficiency, while the U.S. ranked 72nd
in that category. Overall, Oman ranked 8th, while the U.S. ranked
37th. I was anxious to see what one of the top ranked healthcare
systems in the world looked like, especially since it ranked almost
thirty positions higher than the U.S. The difference between what
I expected, and what I saw first-hand, became a defining junc-
ture for me. How could the great healthcare system of the U.S. be
ranked so much lower than countries that I instinctively knew, and
was later to prove, could not be seriously compared to the U.S?

I knew within hours of being in-country that a new part of
my life was about to open. My Omani education began right away.
On my first night in Muscat, Oman's capital, I was introduced to
one of the Royal physicians, a learned Indian cardiologist who had
trained in the U.K. and had been made a citizen of Oman by HM
Sultan Qaboos. I learned of His Majesty's bloodless palace coup

overthrowing his father, the reigning monarch, in 1970; and of the continuing Omani Renaissance under HM who is known for his love of family, the power of education, music, and most of all, his people.

I spent a week in Oman touring, lecturing, and learning about their healthcare system with unfettered access. After coming to know many of Oman's citizens, I began to understand their global reputation for friendliness. This characteristic undoubtedly arose out of necessity to help them get along with the many visitors that have passed through that crossroads of Asia and Europe over the ages. There were the merchants who followed the Spice routes between the Mediterranean and Egypt in the West, and India and China in the East. Of course, there were the many invaders that Oman was also famous for. Today, you can tour a multitude of spectacular Omani forts, whose complexity and weight of fortifications are clear reminders that Oman is also famous for the finest architects and engineers. In addition, there is one of the most famous substances in Christendom which is grown today only in Islamic Oman: frankincense. It is famous as being the most savory form of frankincense, indigenous only to one small region of of the Sultanate where the Al Hajar Mountains come close enough to the sea to allow clouds to form along with enough precipitation to be favorable for its' growth.

I was permitted to lecture in and tour every hospital in the region of Oman's capital, Muscat, including the Royal Hospital. Thankfully, there was never a language barrier since everyone spoke English. I asked many questions of hospital administrators (mostly Western trained), local doctors, and government representatives. I was most anxious to see their technical diagnostic and therapeutic capabilities. I asked about their doctors; the number of primary care and specialist physicians; where they went to medical school, trained, and how that information was documented.

I made rounds in the Royal Hospital's Intensive Care Unit (ICU), speaking to many of the attending physicians. I asked to be shown the medical records departments, and inquired about their Healthcare Information Technology (HIT). I was especially interested in visiting the Obstetrical and Pediatric units as well.

Of particular interest, wherever I traveled around Oman, I asked almost everyone that I met including taxi drivers and store clerks (usually expats from India or Pakistan), in addition to Omani citizens and various well-healed residents, what they would do if they or a family member became seriously ill. Almost without exception, they quickly answered that they would fly to the U.S. or UK if they could; otherwise to India. (Plans for Dubai's Healthcare City on which I was a consultant at the behest of Dubai's Ruler, HH. Sheikh Mohammed bin Rashid Al Maktoum, had not yet been announced.) It was clear that the Sultanate was exporting their sicker patients. These factors, I was sure, would skew the findings of the WHO ranking.

8. RESULTS OF MY FACT FINDING*

In 1975, His Majesty Qaboos bin Said Al Said, Sultan of Oman (HM), initiated a Healthcare Renaissance by a Royal Decree in which he assured the citizens that healthcare was a fundamental right, which would be extended free-of-charge to all.[19] By the time of my first visit in 2002, improvement in the healthcare system had been impressive, and indicative of a true healthcare Renaissance. In 1970, there were only two hospitals in Oman, but by 2000 there were fifty-four. [19]

Over the succeeding decade, modernization of the Omani Health System has included a process of "Omanization," building a healthcare workforce of doctors (primary and specialists) and nurses through in-country training with expected goals extending well beyond 2020. In 2004, the Ministry of Health launched an Oman Medical Specialty Board to certify medical school graduates as well as post-graduate residency programs modeled after those in the U.S. [20] In 2004, a smart card Healthcare Information Technology was launched for its 2.7 million citizens.[21]

Despite its impressive development, the Omani Healthcare system could not be considered as a top world leader by any modern criteria except those espoused by collectivist nations, and entities such as the WHO*. Oman could not be compared to any country in the developed world, and was only average, in my view, among those in the developing world.

It was clear that the WHO wished to send a message that would advance its' hidden, collectivist, agenda. The WHO study rewarded or punished member countries by ranking them based on the intent of their Ministries of Health, or other controlling entities, to ultimately develop Universal Healthcare systems, and to contribute funds to a general, prepaid cash pool to be used at its discretion without notifying the parent country.[22]

THE WHO WORLD REPORT 2000 RANKING SYSTEM

The rankings[23] are based on an index of the following factors:

- Health: disability-adjusted life expectancy (50%)
- Responsiveness: speed of service, protection of privacy (25%)
- Fair financial contribution (25%)

COLLECTIVISM IN THE WHO 2000 REPORT

In the world ranking, Oman was placed first based on performance of health systems, and eighth in overall performance amongst the 191 member states of World Health Organization. When we consider the many medical centers, medical specialists and availability to diagnostic and other bio-medical technology in the U.S, on a common sense level, this designation does not ring true.

However, the WHO vision includes "placing health at the cen-

ter of the broader development agenda." To that aim, the WHO
includes all entities of financing, regulation, and provision of health
actions whose primary intent is to improve or maintain health.
Criteria of primary intent has been replaced with an expanded
definition of the health system, including efforts to improve road
and vehicle safety as well as personal health services whether they
contribute to health or not. [24, 25]

In its stated goal to redistribute wealth within each country and member state, the WHO has undertaken a comprehensive collectivist approach where those member states with
the most money, or are the most developed, contribute the
most to other member countries through financial transfers.
According to Twila Brase of the Citizen's Council of Health
Freedom, the WHO report promotes centralized collection
and pooling in order to further the goal of redistribution. And,
in order to enforce the necessary limits on healthcare services,
the report suggests that physicians and other practitioners be
monitored through the process of data collection, and if necessary be sanctioned for communicating unnecessary or im-
permissible information to patients, noting that practitioners
are difficult to control. The WHO advocates the creation of
a national benefit package with lists of available healthcare
treatments. The lists, coupled with practitioner-controlled
mechanisms such as clinical protocols, registration, training,
and licensing and accreditation processes, can then be used
to enforce healthcare rationing. Could these tactics that in-
fringe on provider liberty become part of the ACA? Many are
already being considered. [26]

Individualism, a most precious American principle is, by definition, the opposite of collectivism. We regard the individual as a
complete moral entity compared to the 'group' in collectivist models. In healthcare, that philosophy translates to a specific loss of
liberty. In collectivist healthcare systems, individuals with rare disorders are afforded little or no healthcare support. The collectivist

standard is a perversion of the Judeo-Christian principle that every life is sacred. Thus, assets 'squandered' on individuals deny the group that may harbor disorders that are more common. Implied is an explicit choice of priorities where rationing may be necessary for individuals, in order to favor the group.

Under the guise of fairness, collectivist governments with universal healthcare systems control production and distribution in order to make certain that common disorders and high prevalence problems get funded, while those with rare disorders often have little or no funding.27 One worry in this regard is the potential that the Independent Payment Advisory Board (IPAB), through its' ability to place a global cap on Medicare, and make selective payment reductions, might become the vehicle to pursue this strategy via the ACA.

COMPARISON OF U.S. HEALTHCARE WITH NATIONALIZED SYSTEMS

THE UNITED KINGDOM NATIONAL HEALTH SERVICE (BEVERIDGE SYSTEM)

Great Britain's National Health Service (NHS) was established in 1948 and provides health care to all British residents. It is referred to as the Beveridge Model (named after the British economist, William Beveridge).

9. COSTS

"The system is financed largely (about 83%) through tax payments just like the police force or the public library. In Britain, you never get a doctor bill. The low costs are determined by the government, which is the sole payer controlling all doctors' services and fees. Consultants are specialists, and patients must be referred by the General Practitioner gatekeepers." [28] [29]

The NHS, like all the nationalized systems, keeps its health care expenditures relatively low while providing universal access to health care at a high cost: rationing of care through imposition of what Americans would deem unacceptable waiting times. Though patients have relatively easy access to primary and emergency care, specialty care is rationed through long waiting lists and a limit on the availability of new technologies.

Management of the degree of financial expenditures of the system is purposely regulated by varying access to care resulting in attrition through postponements and well-understood patterns of death. Often, services are simply not provided. Queuing lines have become the symbol for nationalized health systems. The NHS devotes considerable resources to high-return services such as prenatal and infant care. Diseases occurring less frequently receive disproportionately less funding. They become the losers in the collectivist system.

Funding for the NHS Mental Health Services has been lowered to crisis proportions. Even excessive taxation is incapable of fully funding needed services because of historic drastic cuts. Recent moderate funding increases stimulated long waiting times for in-hospital beds, especially for children, as well as for outpatient psychotherapy. [30]

Rationing through waiting, and serial reduction in services, are no longer tolerated in the UK. Ironically, the NHS is undergoing a broad movement toward privatization in order to relieve the stresses on the system. The very programs that so many Progressives and outright collectivists are pushing America into, has been largely discredited in England. [31] [32] [33]

10. ACCESS IS DECEPTIVE*

Access to the NHS is deceptive. Although they purport to make it equal, it is not so. In comparing the delivery of services between the U.S. and the UK NHS, the UK system lacks in several serious ways. The concise way to describe that difference is that the NHS makes choices that deviate from American values of equality and freedom of choice. The NHS openly rations services through delay (waiting lists). Their strategy for equitable provision of care is to devote considerable resources to high-return services such as prenatal and infant care, while limiting access to care for more expensive procedures through postponement (waiting), or simply not providing selected services. Since private insurance is available, evidence shows that upper-class patients have received substantially more care for a given illness than have lower-class patients. Rationed care cuts monetary costs, and even with increased expenditures from the healthcare reforms, total U.K. expenditures are expected to be well below the European Union and the United States. A wait list of 1 million people has become the hallmark of the UK system.

The NHS is lauded for improving the wait for specialist appointments since the NHS Plan was published in 2000, when nearly 500,000 people waited longer than three months just to see a specialist. However, according to late 2007 data, 30,832 were still waiting more than twenty-six weeks just to receive diagnostic tests, including 16,551 who had waited more than a year. Even now, almost 15 percent of patients in England still wait more than a full month after seeing a general practitioner for a specialist appointment so they can take the next step toward diagnosis and treatment.

The NHS is a collectivist healthcare system. Its inherent methods would be inconsistent with America's first principles. Claims of 'equality' do not mean equal rights for all. Provision of medical services are unequally distributed to patients with considerable resources to high-return services such as prenatal and infant care, while limiting access to care for more expensive procedures-through postponement (waiting), or simply not providing selected services. The NHS provides equal access to citizens who happen to require high-return system services, but not so to patients in

need of more expensive, specialized care. These patients are subjected to long waits that, at best, 'costs' time, loss of productivity
and happiness. At worst, a patient may die unnecessarily during
the inordinant waiting period. Services may not be offered at all
by the NHS if it is too expensive, and no payment is provided to
travel to other locales where treatments are readily available. However, since private insurance is available in the UK to those who
can afford it, access is being denied to lower income consumers in
what then becomes a two-tiered healthcare system. [37] [38] [39] [40] [41]

Performance Under the NHS

- Americans have better survival rates than Europeans for common cancers.
- Americans have better access to treatment for chronic di
  eases than patients do in other developed countries.
- Americans spend less time waiting for care than patients in
  the United Kingdom.
- Americans have better access to important new technologies
  such as medical imaging than do patients in Britain do.[34]

QUALITY OF SERVICES MEASURED BY CONSUMER SATISFACTION.

If government-controlled nationalized health systems were the
"utopia" that they were purported to be, why would more than 70
percent of German, Canadian, Australian, New Zealand, and British citizens believe that their system needed "fundamental change"
or "complete rebuilding," or need "urgent" reform?[34]

The public's opinion, often an accurate reflection of health
care quality, seems to have demonstrated that nationalized systems
were not highly thought of by the citizens who used them. And,
even more telling, in 1989, as a result of widespread public dissatisfaction, the British government began dismantling its National
Health Service, and reintroduced market-based health care competition.[35] Compare those figures to the eighty percent of Americans
who say they are satisfied with the quality of their health care. In

fact, the overwhelming majority of Americans, about threefourths, are happy with their current healthcare coverage. [36] Is that consistent with the far-flung calls that America's healthcare system is a scandalous failure, and it is urgent enough that we fix it now?

THE GERMAN NATIONAL HEALTH SERVICE SICKNESS FUND (BISMARCK SYSTEM) [28 34 37]

The Bismarck System was named for the Prussian Chancellor Otto von Bismarck, who invented the welfare state as part of the unification of Germany in the 19th century. Despite its European heritage, this system of providing healthcare would look fairly familiar to Americans.

The basic approach is mandatory enrollment in an insurance system referred to as 'sickness funds.' Health insurance is mandatory for all working people in Germany, with costs being shared equally between employer and employee. Employee shares are drawn as payroll taxes at a rate of approximately 14.3 percent. Sickness funds provide a comprehensive set of benefits which also provide disability insurance to those not working because of illness. Outpatient provider services are paid on a fee-for-service basis, and payment for hospital care is deferred on a later time. In the German system, both public and private hospitals exist, with the public using salaried physicians about 50% of the time. Hospital operating expenses are covered by sickness funds and capital expenses are covered by the state. [28]

As a counterbalance, most private physicians generally do not admit patients to the hospital. Instead, many doctors have invested in well-equipped, outpatient facilities that compete with hospitals to provide a wide variety of ambulatory procedures.

Challenges to German System:

The German System is currently facing several serious challenges that may impact on its ability to maintain services at current rates. The first is that the aging of the German population along with high unemployment rates have narrowed the base for payroll contributions to the funds. Those with private insurance have begun to opt for other choices resulting in their sickness funds in some instances not covering the statutory programs. Co-payments at the point of service have become required in many instances. [28]

THE CANADIAN NATIONAL HEALTHCARE SYSTEM (HYBRID NHS)

The Canadian system is itself a hybrid, with elements of both the Beveridge and Bismarck systems. [28] Payment comes from a government-run insurance program that every citizen pays into. Public funds account for more 70% of total health spending. Lack of marketing expenses tends to keep this payment under control.

In Canada, coverage must be universal, comprehensive, and portable, meaning that individuals can transfer their coverage to other provinces as they migrate across the country.

Most Canadian physicians are in private practice and have hospital admitting privileges. They are reimbursed by the provinces on a fee-for-service basis under fee schedules negotiated by the provincial governments and their professional societies.

The Canadian system appears to be more effective than the U.S. system in several respects:[28]

THE REAL COSTS OF THE CANADIAN NATIONAL HEALTHCARE SYSTEM (HYBRID NHS)

Fee for service costs are lower, and financial barriers do not exist. Health status as measured by mortality rates is superior and Canadians have longer life expectancies and lower infant mortality rates than do U.S. residents.

These are some of the features that collectivists point out when touting nationalized healthcare over the our previous system built upon American values. But what they fail to point out is the real cost of that system.

The *real* cost to Canadians of their 'free' healthcare is heavy taxation, rationing of care and under-performance of their health-care delivery system. In 2013, a typical Canadian family of four can expect to pay $11,320 for public health care insurance.

Canadian families pay for healthcare through the tax system. That high price buys them long wait times and lack of medical technologies compared to the American system. In fact, Canada's healthcare system is the developed world's most expensive universal-access health care program and, it is getting more expensive. Before inflation, the cost of public health care insurance went up by 53.3 per cent over the last decade. Changing demographics mean Canada's healthcare system has a funding gap of $537 billion.

The expensive healthcare system's under-performance is thanks to 7% annual increases on healthcare spending during the period 2004-2010, which also had the impact of reducing bio-medical research funding which resulted in reduced innovations.

UNDERPERFORMANCE

Wait times in Canada are among the longest in the developed world. It may take 3-6 months to get an appointment with a specialist, plus 2 or more months for a diagnostic CT or MRI, and even more time waiting for surgery. Doctors in Canada don't have access to the same technology their US counterparts.

One published case report demonstrates the impact of this problem: "The reason my biopsy came back inconclusive is that the doctor at Mt. Sinai did not have the benefit of ultrasound guidance when he stuck the needle in my neck 4-5 times in 2004. He therefore missed the tumor. At MD Anderson Cancer Center in Houston (where I went since "indefinite" seemed too long a wait), they did an ultrasound-guided biopsy which hit the tumor the first time. If Canadian docs had access to the basic technology needed to do their jobs, I suspect patient care would be better and more accurate, wait times would decline, and rework and therefore costs would decline."[42] Canadians are thus faced with the following options to cope with their increased burdens:

- Find new sources of tax revenue,
- Impose more stringent fee and budgetary controls on health
- providers,
- Find ways to increase efficiency in health care delivery,
- Scale back on benefits by no longer insuring some previously covered services, and impose user fees.

Canada has Universal access alright. But its cost forces the question "Access to what?" This is exactly what Americans face under the ACA.

DO YOU STILL WANT A NATIONALIZED HEALTH-CARE SYSTEM [37] [34]

We now see that what amounts to under-funding of the Canadian Health System can cause long wait periods for hospital services due to limits on hospital capacity and availability of biotechnology equipment.

The waiting and queues found in Canada would be unacceptable to many U.S. patients. That there is a greater level of amenities in the United States, and a greater availability of specialized care, and high-tech medicine, is often viewed as an indication of superior quality care.

In delaying access to cancer specialists, "Late diagnosis was almost certainly a major contributor to poor survival in England for three of the most prevalent cancers (breast, colorectal and lung)" and "between 5,000 and 10,000 deaths within five years of diagnosis could be avoided every year if efforts to promote earlier diagnosis and appropriate primary surgical treatment are successful."

Roughly 75 percent of referrals to a specialist are generated by the family doctor,[11] after which Canadians wait weeks to months to see a specialist. Overall statistics from Statistics Canada show that 45.6 percent wait less than one month, while 40.5 percent wait from one to three months, and about 14 percent wait more than three months to see the specialist, before being placed on the waiting list for treatment, if needed. By illness, about 41 percent of those with heart disease or stroke, 43 percent with cancer, 54 percent with cataracts, 55 percent with asthma, 58 percent with a skin disorder, 61 percent with a gynecological condition, and 81 percent with arthritis wait more than one month for their doctor appointment to even determine if treatment is needed.

In Ontario, Canada, those with pain requiring possible hip or knee replacement, wait an average of eleven weeks before seeing a specialist, and the majority wait more than nine months for the actual surgery. [12] For those with gastrointestinal disorders, total wait times from primary care referral to specialist investigationwere "protracted relative to CAG (Canadian Association of Gastroenterology) consensus recommendations, regardless of whether patients were considered to require urgent investigation (suspected cancer of GI bleeding) or not."

Single-payer health insurance systems are a form of Nationalized Systems where the government pays all the medical bills (Canada).

However, comparative performance benchmarks show:

- US system is more egalitarian than the Canadian system,
- Uninsured Americans get as much as or more preventive carethan insured Canadians (such as mammograms, PSAtests, colonoscopies),
- Low-income whites in the United States are in better health than low-income whites in Canada.
- Although minorities do less well in both countries, we treat our minority populations better than the Canadians do, and even though thousands of people in both countries go to

hospital emergency rooms for care they can't get anywhere else, people in our emergency rooms are treated more quickly and with better results than people in Canadian emergency rooms.

Perhaps the most important fact that I emphasize in this book, is that while it has its flaws, the U.S. healthcare system must be seen for what it is: the best in the world, even unrivaled, based upon its history and the fact-based statistics. Once U.S. healthcare can be examined objectively, I believe that most reformers will seek to restore its' exceptionalism along lines set forth by America's first principles.

REFERENCES

1. Professional Licensure Beginning in 1867 http://mises.org/journals/jls/3_1/3_1_5.pdf

2. https://www.aamc.org/newsroom/reporter/170142/medical_education_standards.html

3. http://pdf.usaid.gov/pdf_docs/PNABQ044.pdf)(Quality Assurance Methodology Refinement Series Licensure, Accreditation, and Certification:Approaches to Health Services Quality, Anne L. Rooney, R.N., M.S., M.P.H. Paul R. van Ostenberg, D.D.S., M.S. Aprill 1999

4. Sultz, Harry A.; Young, Kristina M. (2010-08-23). Health Care USA (p. 100). Jones & Bartlett Learning. Kindle Edition

5. Atlas, Scott W. (2012-01-03). In Excellent Health: Setting the Record Straight on America's Health Care (Hoover Institution Press Publication) (Kindle Locations 3448-3450). Chicago Distribution. Kindle Edition. (Kindle Locations 3440-3441). (Kindle Locations 3445-3447). (Kindle Locations 3431-3440)

6. Murray, C.J.L., A WHO Framework for Health System Performance Assessment. , pp.1–27.

7. Scott W Atlas, 04.01.2011. The Worst Study Ever ? Commentary Magazine, http://www.commentarymagazine.com/article/the-worst-study-ever/

8. http://en.wikipedia.org/wiki/World_Health_Organization_ranking_of_health_systems_in_2000#Ranking

9. Health Systems: Improving Performance, WHO, ORT, E.P., 2000.

10. Tanner, M., 2007. The Grass is Not Always Greener: A Look at National Health Care Systems Around the World, Policy Anaysis, www.cato.org/pubs/pas/pa-613.pdf

11. Vincente Navarro, Scott Atlas, Joseph S. Coyne, DrPH and Peter Hilsenrath, http://www.ncbi.nlm.nih.gov/pmc/articles/PMC1447380/

12. Philip Musgrove, PhD. Editor-in-Chief of the WHO 2000 Report, in The Lancet, 2003

13. McKee, M., 2010. The World Health Report 2000: 10 years on. Health policy and planning, 25(5), pp.346–8. Available at: http://www.ncbi.nlm.nih.gov/pubmed/20798126 [Accessed May 19, 2013]

14. WHO's Hidden Agenda (Published in Ideas on Liberty by the Foundation for Economic Education) by Twila Brase October 2000 http://www.cchfreedom.org/cchf.php/173#.UuR34hDTldh

15. The Worst Study Ever ? Scott W Atlas, Commentary Magazine, 2011. April, 2011 http://www.commentarymagazine.com/article/the-worst-study-ever/

16. Assessment of the World Health Report 2000 Vicente Navarro, THE LANCET • Vol 356 • November 4, 2000

17. http://www.freedomworks.org/content/health-care-not-right-o

18. http://www.who.int/whr/2000/en/whr00_en.pdf

19. CHALLENGING HEALTH CARE SYSTEM SUSTAINABILITY IN OMAN, Ali A. Al Dhawi, Ph.D, FACHE,

20. Futaisi, A. Al et al., Physician Training & Certification In Oman.

21. Sultanate, T. & Id, N., 2002. Development of the Solution. , pp.1–5. CASE STUDY 'The Sultanate of Oman – National ID Program'

22. http://www.who.int/whr/2010/10_chap03_en.pdf

23. WHO World Health Report 2000 Rankings Wiki

24. A WHO Framework for Health System Performance Assessment Christopher JL MurrayJulio Frenk Evidence and Information for Policy World Health Organization http://www.who.int/healthinfo/paper06.pdf

25. WORLD HEALTH ORGANIZATION (WHO): STRATEGY ON MEASURING RESPONSIVENESS Charles Darby, et al. http://www.who.int/healthinfo/paper23.pdf and (http://www.who.int/responsiveness/en/.

26. WHO's Hidden Agenda Published in Ideas on Liberty by the Foundation for Economic Education October 2000 by Twila Brase

27. http://thepatientfactor.com/canadian-health-care-information/universal-health-care-who-says-its-the-fairest-of-them-all/

28. www.udel.edu/Economics/clink/London/comparative.ppt

29. Health Care USA Understanding Its Organization and Delivery Seventh Edition Harry A. Sultz, DDS, MPH; Young, Kristina M. (2010-08-23). Health Care USA (p. i). Jones & Bartlett Learning. Kindle Edition.

30. http://www.commonwealthfund.org/~/media/Files/Publications/Fund%20 Report/2013/Nov/1717_Thomson_intl_profiles_hlt_care_sys_2013_v2.pdf

31. https://www.opendemocracy.net/ournhs/paul-evans/race-to-privatise-en-glands-nhs

32. http://www.hulldailymail.co.uk/NHS-privatisation-fears-Health-share-wins-pound-8/story-22049360-detail/story.html

33. http://pureoai.bham.ac.uk/ws/files/10884391/Privatizing_the_English_Na-tional_Health_Service.pdf

34. Tanner, M., 2007. The Grass is Not Always Greener: A Look at National Health Care Systems Around the World. http://www.cato.org/sites/cato. org/files/pubs/pdf/pa-613.pdf

35. National Health Insurance: A Medical Disaster : The Freeman : Founda-tion for Economic Education fee.org · by JARRET B. WOLLSTEIN · October 1, 1992

36. CNN/Opinion Research Corp. poll, March 2009; Gallup poll, 2007, 2006, 2005, 2004, 2003, 2002, 2001; Quinnipiac University poll, October 2007.

37. Atlas, S.W., 2009. Here's a second opinion. The Journal of the Oklahoma State Medical Association, 102(8), p.275. Available at: http://www.ncbi. nlm.nih.gov/pubmed/19750819 . Scott W. Atlas is the David and Joan Trai-tel Senior Fellow at the Hoover Institution, and senior fellow by courtesy at the Freeman Spogli Institute for International Studies at Stanford.

38. Martin Beckford, "Patients Struggle Even to Get on NHS Waiting Lists," Telegraph, July 29, 2011, http://www.telegraph.co.uk/health/health-news/8671127/Patients-struggle-even-to-get-on-NHS-waiting-lists.html .

39. Oliver Wright, "Cataracts, Hips, Knees and Tonsils: NHS Begins Ra-tioning Operations: Almost Two-thirds of Trusts Affected as Cuts Bite," Independent, July 28, 2011,http://www.independent.co.uk/life-style/ health-and-families/health-news/cataracts-hips-knees-and-tonsils-nhs-be-gins-rationing-operations-2327268.html.

40. Jenny Hope, "Cancer Operations Are Denied to Thousands of Elderly Patients 'Because of Ageism,'" MailOnline, March 19, 2011, http://www. dailymail.co.uk/health/article-1367781/Cancer-operations-denied-thou-sands-elderly-patients-ageism.html .

41. Pipes, Sally C. (2012-01-09). The Pipes Plan: The Top Ten Ways to Dis-

mantle Obamacare (Kindle Locations 2554-2568). Regnery Publishing. Kindle Edition.

42. Canada's healthcare system expensive and underperforming, Talking Now Supporting Canadians with voice problems heathertalks • April 27, 2013 •

* Among my conclusions were:

Insufficient licensure verification• Insufficient board certification No accreditation of medical schools (In 2002 Sultan Qaboos Medical School not yet accredited (2012)Sultan Qaboos University Med J, November 2012, Vol. 12, Iss. 4, pp.406-410, Epub. 20th • lack of specialists HIT smart cards (Five million card for two million citizens) (OMAN had no ID no Identity card until 2004-200five. Imaging healthcare with no means of proving ID. Many multiples of2.five millions (populations) were issued at hospitals every time people went to differentfacility where registration cards were issued) Journal of Health Sciences Management and Public HealthCHALLENGING HEALTH CARE SYSTEM-SUSTAINABILITY IN OMAN[1] University of Scranton, USA[2] Ph.D., FACHE, FACMPE, FAAMA, Universityof Scranton, USA.Ali A. Al Dhawii, Daniel J. West, Jr. [2] ABSTRACT

The healthcare system in Oman is being reformed. During last three decades, the systemhas demonstrated and reported great achievements in health care services, preventive andcurative medicine. In 2001, WHO ranked Oman first because of what was described as a"spectacular performance" in reducing infant mortality rate over the past three decades. Thehealthcare system in Oman is facing a challenge of sustainability of achievement. In this paper, current health status indicators are presented along with effort to maintain healthoutcomes. Threats of sustainability are identified and international financing approaches arereviewed to develop a model for sustaining reform in Oman

CHAPTER SIX:

HEALTHCARE SYSTEMS

There has been much discussion about the degree of impact that the ACA has had on the U.S. healthcare system. Some say that the law primarily changed the health insurance structure but little else. However, as I demonstrate in this book, its effects are far-reaching, encompassing every aspect of healthcare delivery, as well as its supporting sub-systems. In order to illustrate this, we examine the component parts of healthcare systems in general, and pre-2010 U.S. healthcare in particular.

The primary intent of any healthcare system is to preserve a population's 'health'.[1] It is the healthcare delivery system, a sub-set of the overall healthcare system that carries out healthcare's primary functions. However, there are three other basic functions of healthcare systems that must maintain their own integrity and sustainability in order to support healthcare delivery: 1) financing of the system, 2) insurance coverage for the consumers, and 4) payment to providers and vendors.[1]

The massive healthcare industry grew out of a need to support the primary intent of healthcare, to deliver care. However America's healthcare system is without rival. It seems impossible, however, to assign a degree of exceptionalism to the overall healthcare system would prove impossible. Our enormous healthcare system was, in fact, "so complicated that no one person [could] ever fully grasp everything that is going on. As individuals, all we ever really see is a small slice of the system" as described by John C. Goodman in his book, "Priceless: Curing the Healthcare Crisis." Most typical U.S. patients might only see their doctor several times a year, and possibly undergo some routine outpatient laboratory or imaging studies. What they may be unaware of is the enormous environment of multiple systems functioning all around them. It is so large, that the annual total Health Spending in 2014 was projected to have risen to over $3.1 trillion, or $9,697 per person, and a Health Care as Share of GDP of 18.3%, making the American healthcare system, in and of itself, the 5th largest economy in the world—larger than the entire budget of France. Medical care in the United States is an enormous industry that includes thousands of independent medical practices, partnerships and provider organizations, public and private, for-profit and nonprofit corporations and institutions such as hospitals, nursing homes, and other specialized care facilities. The federal, state, and local governments are all integral elements of the healthcare system. Healthcare is by far the largest service industry in the country. There can be no doubt that this extended network of systems is by nature unwieldy and unmanageable, in need of constant cycles of vigilance and reforms. Hence, the overall goal of reform should be to maintain the highest possible level of functionality of the supporting healthcare systems so to enable exceptional delivery of its primary functions, the diagnosis, treatment, and prevention of disease. [2] [3] [4]

America found itself with a superb medical delivery system enveloped by an enormous healthcare Leviathan, a biblical sea creature that symbolizes a system too complex to assure optimal access to care for everyone, too disorganized to prevent a multitude of institutional and professional mistakes that result in death, disabilities and suffering, and a system too inefficient to maintain cost-effectiveness. Our healthcare delivery system prior to 2010, whose major elements had undergone a century of achievement, was in need of significant reform aimed at becoming a consolidated, modern, set of systems, each fully accountable and inter-operable, and driven by the all of its' stakeholders who had, to date, been stifled by over-regulation and government meddling.

TWO WORLDVIEWS, TWO FORMS OF HEALTHCARE

There are many variations in the way the basic functions of healthcare systems can be organized. Any component part of the system may be more or less important from system to system. In addition, the central organizing principles from which systems are developed also vary greatly. The system must fit the purpose for which it was proposed, and then the principles behind its development must become widely disseminated. [5]

Healthcare systems can be organized around cultural beliefs as they do in the U.S. healthcare system. Our healthcare system was based upon beliefs in America's First Principles which have continuously served as the sustaining force of exceptionalism, suggesting therefore that those values should act as bases of reform.

Two opposing belief systems, or worldviews, provide the basis for healthcare systems as envisioned by two historical medical greats who each spoke to their concept of healthcare reform based upon their societies' cultures and needs for reform. One was the German pathologist, Rudolf Virchow [6] who lived from 1821 to 1902, and famously said: "Medicine is a social science, and politics nothing but medicine at a larger scale" [6] His analysis, coming during a severe epidemic, emphasized the multiple social and cultural factors involved in healthcare reform at that time. Instead of recommending medical changes (i.e., more doctors or hospitals), he outlined a revolutionary program of social reconstruction, including the radical step of disestablishment of the Catholic Church. The Medical Reform Movement of 1848 was influenced by him, and traces of his influence on the subsequent development of social medicine remain today.

That quotation would suggest that Virchow would have approved of the collectivist healthcare system that would later be introduced in Germany by its ruler, Otto von Bismarck, in the 1880's.[7] Bismarck introduced the world's first welfare state, which included the collectivist national social health insurance. Collectivism is the idea that the individual's life belongs not to him but to the group or society of which he is merely a part; that he has no individual rights, and that he must sacrifice his values and goals for the group's "greater good." According to collectivism, the group or society is the basic unit of moral concern, and the individual is of value only insofar as he serves the group. Collectivism is a basic cultural element that exists as the reverse of individualism in human nature. [8]

It would come as no surprise to learn that the other opposing medical great to whom I refer, who would extol individualism in human nature, was William Osler. He recognized that "variability is the law of life, and as no two faces are the same, so no two bodies are alike, and no two individuals react alike and behave alike under the abnormal conditions we know as disease" [9]

American medicine recognizes Osler's fundamental principles, and rejects the practice of "one-size-fits-all."[10] Traditionally, doctors take detailed histories from their patients in an effort to elucidate specific facts about the patient that separates him/her from all others. Personalized data help not only to differentiate possible diseases that lie at the root of patients' symptoms, but also to devise individualized, specific courses of treatment that would be more effective than a single, conventional treatment. Modern doctors seek to apply personalized medicine by custom-tailoring treatments to individual patients. Further, we are now on the cusp of the most significant technological and clinical achievements since the Hopkins experiment; so great as to be capable of fulfilling William Osler's greatest aspirations: modern genetic medicine. Biomedical research has yielded the capability to inexpensively determine the essential genetic make-up of every person, the ultimate goal of personalized medicine.

VARIATIONS IN HEALTHCARE SYSTEMS BASED UPON FINANCING

Most modern healthcare models are based on their mode of financing which means where and how money comes into the system to pay for it, and how it goes out to pay providers and vendors. Variations may occur within financing models pertaining to what percentage is controlled by private interests, and what percentage is government controlled.

HEALTHCARE SYSTEMS ORGANIZED BY DEGREE OF CENTRAL REGULATION

In Chapter Five, I compared the structures and performance of three nationalized healthcare systems (The Beveridge Model (UK), The Bismarck Model (Germany), The National Health Insurance Hybrid Model (Canada)) that are characterized as being centrally regulated, with a single-payer.

THE U.S. HEALTHCARE SYSTEM

In 2009, prior to passage of the ACA, federal, state, and local governments accounted for more than 60 percent of all U.S. healthcare system spending. [11] The new healthcare reform law completely changed the degree of control by government.

After the enactment of the ACA, the U.S. healthcare, federal-private hybrid system has become far more heavily weightedtoward government control. Under the ACA, the private sector's share of healthcare spending is reduced to 33 percent, with public financing making up the rest. Most of the 33 percent is represented by government-regulated private insurance in the ACA insurance exchanges. While the government lacks 100 percent control over healthcare, its intervention is expansive. The ACA expands existing federal programs, the largest being Medicaid in order to cover millions of mostly low-income and uninsured people. It establishes new subsidies, many new taxes, and new regulatory agencies that influence all public and private insurance, and extends to the regulation of consumers, choices of physicians, as well as to dictate how doctors practice medicine regardless of patients' mode of insurance. The federal government will have control over your care. Sec. 1311 of the law empowers the Secretary of Health and Human Services [12], to dictate how doctors treat privately insured patients and what questions patients can be asked, including their role in the doctor-patient relationship. [13][14]

Government funding comes through income taxes and taxes paid by workers as a percentage of their wages, from fees paid for by individuals mandated to purchase coverage, and through private state-based insurance exchanges for employees and their families, with contributions to be paid for by an employer mandate set to partially begin in 2015.[15] Governmental expenditures went to Hospital Care, Physician and Clinical Services, Dental Services, Home Health Care, Nursing Care Facilities and Continuing Care Retirement Communities Durable Medical Equipment (long-lasting medical products including beds, wheelchairs, Oxygen canisters, and many more).

A NEW MODEL OF HEALTHCARE BASED UPON A PROGRESSIVE'S WORLDVIEW

In 1991, the WHO adapted a new, more inclusive model of healthcare system. Developed by, Milton Roemer, MD, MA (Sociology), a self-proclaimed socialist, "Roemer viewed the Soviet Union as embodying a vision of the future, with a health system more oriented to preventive than curative medicine built on principles of equity." [16][17][18] The chief organizing principle of the WHO system was to include "all the activities whose primary purpose was to promote, restore or maintain health." [19] This definition signaled that the system would cross "boundaries of health into activities that have secondary health-enhancing benefits to communities such as safe roads, sanitation, and health equity, which is the equal ability for every member to pay for healthcare expenses." [17] [18] [19] [20] Clearly stated in the "The World Health Report 2000 - Health systems: improving performance" [20], 'equity' was to refer to strategies of redistribution of assets both within each member country, but among countries as well.

The new bio-psychosocial model of health would be greatly expanded to include all activities whose primary purpose it was to promote, restore, or maintain health. [21] This model represented a radical departure from the biomedical model of healthcare combined with humanism described by Sir William Osler. [17] [18] [19] [22] It was 'purpose-built' in order to achieve equal distribution of health devoted resources among its 191 member states, including financing. [19] [23] [24]

The provision to redistribute funds from more wealthy states to be used directly for healthcare for poverty-stricken children, was actually deceitful, covering-up the WHO's hidden agenda to 'shakedown' the wealthier member states for assets that would be used to enrich the lives of the well-to-do [25] In the WHO Report 2000, widespread knowledge of the new definition had not yet been disseminated, and when results of the report were released, it opened the U.S. healthcare system to an unfair campaign of criticism and disinformation that was used to damage its' reputation among member states. Even its Editor-in-Chief was compelled to apologize in scientific journals not only for the failure to prepare member countries for the unexpected and unwarranted outcomes, but also for his malfeasance of data collection and analysis, as well as biased conclusions.

When other governments undertake such redistributive efforts, Americans have the right to understand where the money is going and for what purpose. They have the right to choose how their property is being used, a right spelled out in America's first principles. To rationalize their position, the WHO "dismiss[es] real fairness, the ethic inherent in earning , keeping, and controlling the fruits of one's own labors in exchange for a perverted description of fairness that fits their own need for control." [25]

STAKEHOLDERS IN HEALTHCARE SYSTEMS

Stakeholders are people or organizations that have a vested interest in a healthcare system, and are therefore interested in its' major changes, outcomes and direction. Each of these stakeholders has its' self-interests as well as unique roles in ensuring successful quality improvement. [4]

Primary Stakeholders— patients, doctors, and other healthcare providers who represented the front line participants in medical delivery system.

Secondary Stakeholders--essential in the healthcare system but do not directly deal with patient care. They include government agencies, hospital systems, pharmaceutical companies, pharmacies, and healthcare insurance companies.

Peripheral Stakeholders--professional associations, research organizations, administrators of medical education and training facilities.[4]

UNIQUE CHARACTERISTICS OF U.S. HEALTHCARE

The U.S. healthcare system is difficult to categorize, in part because of its multi-centric origins, other than through recognition of the unique characteristics of its' component parts. In addition, with each component vying for predominance in a $3 trillion sea, it is not surprising that the characteristics of each component may have changed over time due to conflict, reform, and in some cases, competition. In performing its' basic functions of providing financing, insurance coverage, delivery of medical care, and providing payment to providers for products and services, the U.S. Healthcare system is composed of an aggregate of many public (governmental) and private sources. This collection of entities does not form a "group of inter-related components working together coherently toward a common goal or purpose" which would define it as a true "system." In fact, the U.S. healthcare system, while often referred to as such, is not a true "system" per se, rather, as Leiyu Shi and Douglas A. Singh describe in their book," Essentials Of The U.S. Health Care System, it is a "system of organizations," or a system of systems. [26]

IMPERFECT MARKET CONDITIONS

U.S. healthcare has been transformed from a quasi-market-based system to one that is stringently controlled by the government rather than by private organizations and individuals.

In a free market, patients (buyers) and providers (sellers) act independently. Patients should be able to choose their provider based on price and quality. For the healthcare market to be free, unrestrained competition must occur among providers, based on price and quality. A free market requires that patients have information about the availability of various services. In a free market, patients as consumers must directly bear the cost of services received, and make decisions about the purchase of healthcare services. [26]

MEDICAL MALPRACTICE

The U.S. has had a system of compensating patients for professional wrongdoing through medical malpractice insurance (professional liability) when demonstrated through appropriate jurisprudence, a system that has been widely in place since the 1960's, and present in some form since the 1840's.

Every physician must face the ethical dilemma that is medical malpractice. It is not just the impact from the threat, or even the reality of litigation, when a current or past patient, or their family, initiates a suit against you. There is also the understanding that medical malpractice in our society represents an essential form of redress for harm caused to a patient in instances of physician negligence. Doctors also know that adverse events, or untoward incidences that might harm a patient, often due to medical error, occur more frequently than the public is aware, and that close to one-half of the errors were preventable. In a landmark study released in 1999 by the U.S. Institute of Medicine (IOM), "To Err is Human", the nation was shocked to learn that medical errors lead to as many as 98,000 deaths per year.[47]

Another glaring absence in the ACA, in a time where the high cost of medical care is the nation's number one concern, not one line dealing head-on with reform of the medical malpractice system was written into the 2000+ pages of the bill. Unnecessary spending could be reduced with reform of malpractice laws (tort reform). Costs of Malpractice premiums, settlements, and administrative costs are approximately $35 billion, about 2% of total health care costs. Defensive medicine is approximately $66 billion, 3% of total health care costs[28] Implementing all of the listed measures would reduce national premiums for medical liability insurance by about 10%. Therefore, implementation of the proposed measures could lower total health care costs by about 0.5%, or $ 11 billion.

REFERENCES

1. What Is Healthcare System? US healthcare system overview, Foundations of US Health Care Delivery Chapter 2, Shi Singh Singh, D .A . Essentials of the U . S . Health Care System, Second Edition.

2. Goodman, John C. (2012-06-01). Priceless: Curing the Healthcare Crisis (Independent Studies in Political Economy) (pp. 1-2). Independent Publishers Group. Kindle Edition.

3. A supplement to California HealthCare Foundation's Health Care Costs 101, 2014 edition available at www.chcf.org (3) Growth in US Health Care Costs, Emanuel, Ezekiel, Lec. Health Policy and the Affordable Care Act, March 25, 2013, Coursera.org

4. Sultz, Harry A.; Young, Kristina M. (2010-08-23). Health Care USA (Kindle Locations 282-286). Jones & Bartlett Learning. Kindle Edition.

5. J Med Syst. 2003 Oct;27(5):465-73.A theory for classification of health care organizations

6. RUDOLF VIRCHOW AND SOCIAL MEDICINE IN HISTORICAL

PERSPECTIVE Med Hist. Jul 1964; 8(3): 274–278. http://www.ncbi.nlm. nih.gov/pmc/articles/PMC1033391

7. Verh Dtsch Ges Pathol. 2003;87:150-7.

8. http://en.wikipedia.org/wiki/Otto_von_Bismarck#Social_legislation.

9. Heywood, Andrew. Key Concepts in Politics. Palgrave Macmillan. p. 122 in http://en.wikipedia.org/wiki/Collectivism#cite_note-6

10. Personalized medicine: a patient - centered paradigm by Ravinder Mamtani December 1, 2011 ·ncbi.nlm.nih.gov

11. (http://www.forbes.com/sites/chrisconover/2012/08/07/takeover-government-on-track-to-make-up-66-of-healthcare-spending-obamacare/

12. Under Obama Health Care Law: Government-Controlled Private Insurance," Besty McCaughey

13. Full Text - Journal of the American Academy of Psychiatry ...www.jaapl. org/content/40/3/399.full by BK Cooke -2012 -

14. The Doctor–Patient Relationshipwww.ncbi.nlm.nih.gov/...National Center for Biotechnology Information by SD Goold -1999 -

15. Obamacare: Before and After - Discover the Networks www.discoverthe-networks.org/viewSubCategory.asp?id=1957

16. (http://www.ncbi.nlm.nih.gov/pmc/articles/PMC2509620/)

17. Milton I. Roemer Advocate of Social Medicine, International Health, and National Health Insurance Am J Public Health. 2008 September; 98(9): 1596–1597. doi: 10.2105/AJPH.2008.134189 PMCID: PMC2509620

18. Milton I. Roemer Advocate of Social Medicine, International Health, and National Health Insurance Emily K. Abel, PhD, MPH, Elizabeth Fee, PhD, and Theodore M. Brown, PhD, The Meanings of Health and its Promotion,Sartorius, N, Croat Med J. 2006 August; 47(4): 662–664.

19. The Constitution of the World Health Organization. In: World Health Organization: Basic documents. 45th ed. Geneva: World Health Organization; 2005.

20. Rica, C., Salvador, E. & Lucia, S., 2000. WHO 2000 Report derives from: Annex Table 10 Health system performance indexes , estimates for 1997. pp.200–203.

21. A Model for Delivering Psychosocial Health Services - Cancer Care for the Whole Patient - NCBI Bookshelf

22. (http://www.who.int/whr/2000/en/)

23. Am J Psychiatry.1980;137:535–44) (Engel GL. The need for a new medical model: a challenge for biomedicine. Science.1977;196:129–3

24. (The rise and fall of the biopsychosocial model, S. Nassir Ghaemi, MD, MPH, The British Journal of Psychiatry (2009)195: 3-4doi:10.1192/bjp. bp.109.063859)

25. WHO's Hidden Agenda Twila Brase, Published in Ideas on Liberty by the Foundation for Economic Education October 2000 http://www. cchfreedom.org/cchf.php/173#.U_PIHPldVrw

26. Essentials Of The U.S. Health Care System by Leiyu Shi and Douglas A. Singh (Apr 19, 2013), U.S. Healthcare overview 1)

27. Stelfox, H.T . et al., 2006. The "To Err is Human" report and the patient safety literature. Quality & safety in health care.

28. (Brennan, T.A. et al., 1991. SPECIAL ARTICLES INCIDENCE OF ADVERSE EVENTS AND NEGLIGENCE IN HOSPITALIZED PATIENTS Results of the Harvard Medical Practice Study I. , (Appendix I), pp.370–376.) and (Perrin, T., 2007. Investigation of Defensive Medicine in Massachusetts- NCRP. , 2000(November 2008), pp.1–19.) Relations between malpractice claims and adverse events due to negligence. ((SPECIAL ARTICLE, Relation between Malpractice Claims and Adverse Events Due to Negligence — Results of the Harvard Medical Practice Study III A. Russell Localio, J.D., M.P.H., M.S., Ann G. Lawthers, Sc.D., Troyen A. Brennan, M.D., J.D., M.P.H., Nan M. Laird, Ph.D., Liesi E. Hebert, Sc.D., Lynn M. Peterson, M.D., Joseph P. Newhouse, Ph.D., Paul C. Weiler, LL.M., and Howard H. Hiatt, M.D. N Engl J Med 1991; 325:245-251July 25, 1991DOI: 10.1056/NEJM199107253250405).)

CHAPTER SEVEN:

THE IMPACT OF THE ACA

The ACA threatens to deny our freedoms without having any positive impact on healthcare's known weaknesses.

A majority of American's have consistently been opposed to the ACA, both before and after its implementation.[1] And now that we have finally "found out what is in" the bill, most people still don't like it,[2][3] and for good reason. The ACA has removed all choice from healthcare. It has dismantled the best healthcare system in the world, and has failed across the board to deliver on any of the promises that were made to the public in the selling of this law:

Few have been able to keep their health costs and doctors as promised by President Obama. The cost of health insurance premiums are skyrocketing,[4][5] and the cost of healthcare spending continues to rise.[6][7] Medicaid expansion has failed to increase access to healthcare for the poor, and those not covered by health insurance. Healthcare delivery has been disrupted, and has not been made safer or more efficient.*

It is true that millions of newly qualified citizens and residents are now eligible for Medicaid coverage. However, that number is proving to be much lower than was predicted, and not having any effect on health outcomes of the insured. The question remains why less radical solutions to coverage were never considered, and why did the Administration and majority party of both houses of Congress chose to remake one-sixth of the economy when much better, proven alternatives could have been implemented?

The truth is that the intent of the ACA was to transform the country "from a marketplace of ideas, and freedom of choice, to one that is stifled by coercion and mandates," according to Kentucky Senator Paul (REP KY).[8] "The current status of our welfare state demands a clear-thinking American people to recognize that we are in perilous debt, and we cannot sustain costly new entitlements," said news analyst Charles Krauthammer of Fox News. [10] We should now conclude that the ACA must be repealed, and that there is a better way to proceed in order to provide healthcare for the under-privileged without trading in our liberties.

To accept the status quo under the ACA, the U.S. healthcare system would no longer remain a beacon for the rest of the world but would have succumbed to elaborate hoaxes to defraud us of our country's ability to continue to implement its value system. The ACA has already "decimated the best healthcare in the world that was put together as a delicate but operable system." [11]

A number of experts have pointed out that collectivist, single-payer healthcare systems such as those openly favored by Barack Obama [12] put trust in the faceless bureaucrats, [13][14][15] despite the fact that government has consistently proven itself unworthy of that trust, and incapable of running a sustainable healthcare system.[16][17] Just ask our Veterans who are languishing as they wait months and years for appointments that may never come.[18]

Another coercive strategy sure to backfire on ACA architects goes as follows: Changes in the medical education programs will be instituted that are designed to skew medical students and residents away from becoming medical or surgical specialists. ACA decision makers believe that a 10 percent raise in fee reimbursement will incentivize young doctors to choose primary care as a career, and to change their basic philosophy of healthcare management, and become paid gatekeepers for the government. They will be left to face the ire of patients as waiting times expand, and as medical litigation rises, without one line of tort reform relief in the ACA. "Add to this the 30 million extra uninsured, the dramatic growth in the elderly population, and the projected 65,000-doctor shortage predicted for a decade from now, and the responsibility foisted upon the primary care doctors will be overwhelming," says journalist Keith R. Jackson. [18]

These coercive tactics clearly demonstrate that the healthcare reform tactics of the ACA disregard the lessons of history, and disrespect America's first principles. Pumping up the demand of the system should be accompanied by freeing up providers to innovate methods to deal with the problem. Instead, physicians are being forced into boxes that diminish their time and effectiveness with their patients. Physicians should be allowed to exercise their freedoms to use their creativity, including the free-market, to help find innovative solutions to healthcare's weaknesses as well as diseases[19] Doctors are being set-up to deal with too many patients, in too little time to accurately diagnose and treat them in thoughtful, therapeutic, doctor-patient relationships. And, they will have too little knowledge of current medical advances, along with dwindling resources available to help, making primary care medicine impossibly difficult to practice ethically and accurately. Unconscionable waits will go hand in hand with scandalous outcomes, just like they do everywhere national health care takeovers have occurred. [22] [23]

IMPACT OF ACA ON THE HEALTHCARE DELIVERY SYSTEM

American physicians are bracing for the negative impact of the ACA on their practices. Already under tremendous pressure from government regulation and oversight, the profession can now expect to lose even more of its independence and integrity, according to Alyene Senger of the Heritage Foundation. [23]

Authors of the ACA such as Ezekiel Emanuel, view healthcare reform as a battle between out-of-control providers who drive up costs through over-utilization of advanced bio-technical devices, such as C.T. or M.R.I. scanners, injudicious referrals to expensive provider specialists, and choosing to treat patients with expensive, boutique treatments including surgery, when a pill would be just as effective. A 2000 page law has been written to alter that behavior without fixing the fundamental problems underlying healthcare in America.

The thinking behind ACA reform places the government at odds with a physician's intent to practice the best medicine possible. The law intends to reduce costs through coercive containment which means reduction in physician services and salaries, innovation, and the rate of growth of the bio-medical and research industries. Physicians are rightly concerned about their loss of autonomy; that the new law will interfere with their decision making processes, and most of all, come between them and their patient, intruding upon the most clinically important factor to outcome, the doctor-patient relationship. Besides imposing planned annual reimbursement cuts of over 20 percent, doctors also face the need to take care of up to an anticipated 30 million additional Medicaid patients. And since the ACA provides access to these patients by expanding Medicaid, the increased stress on the system will only exacerbate access issues as the supply of doctors will not be able to meet the demand, and talented individuals may be dissuaded from choosing medical training altogether.

According to the Kaiser Family Foundation, "Reduction in reimbursements, combined with increased burdens for the doctors' time, is a perfect formula for professional burnout. In fact, over 214,000 doctors won't participate in the new plans under the Affordable Care Act (ACA,) according to a survey by Medical Group Management Association."[26] These factors give rise to the concern whether doctors, in light of the bureaucratic over-regulation, would continue to practice at all. Rather than fixing healthcare's weaknesses, the ACA no doubt contributes to a crisis that threatens to make things much worse: "The Association of American Medical Colleges has noted that by 2020 we will already need 91,500 more doctors than we are projected to have — 45,000 from primary care and 46,500 surgeons and specialists." [26]

To most doctors, the writing is on the wall: despite their superb medical education, their drive to help their fellow man by making medicine newer and better, they are headed toward mediocrity. The greatest healthcare system ever is being reduced to an ordinary, state-sponsored, public health service in the mold of the Veterans Health Administration.

CONSIDER YOUR NEXT DOCTOR'S APPOINTMENT

It is an unfortunate fact that for each of us, it will take only one event to confer full personal knowledge and experience of virtually every consumer-oriented ill that I refer to in this book. That event does not have to be a serious medical error in your or your loved one's care. It may be far more mundane such as enduring rationing through long waiting times for tests or surgery. or even the cancellation altogether of a test that you have relied on for years that has just been declared 'off plan' because there is not enough evidence to justify the payment. This is exactly what happened with routine mammography for women between age 40-50.[27] Most of us will feel the pain of the dramatic rise in costs that will take place as a result of the ACA's so-called cost containment strategies.

During your next appointment, think about whether you and your doctor have a relationship that could be termed a 'partnership.' Prior to 2010, modern healthcare recognized the importance of making patients central within the therapeutic paradigm (patient 'centeredness') as a means to ethically empower, and enhance such a partnership (the doctor-patient relationship.) In many surveys, the most important element in patient satisfaction is the degree to which such a partnership has taken place. [28] [29] Regardless of your answer, all of that is about to change.

Growing stresses on both parties, many of which are unnecessary, negatively affect outcomes, compliance in chronic and preventive care, and number of hospitalizations, simply by disrupting the doctor-patient relationship, [30] The ACA, will certainly "constrain the freedom of medical providers, limit patient options, and restrict the right of patients to make personal health care decisions in consultation with their doctor." [30]

In any therapeutic relationship, communication and empathy are essential components, having direct effects upon outcomes. No new expensive oral blood glucose lowering agents, or new, sophisticated monitoring devices may be required in order to achieve better control of diabetes, for example. Reduced symptoms from most disorders may not require expensive drugs or prolonged engagement of allied healthcare providers at all. Rather, it appears that when given better relationships with their caregivers, and receiving adequate information on diagnosis and prognosis, most patients experienced better symptom relief and functional outcomes." [29]

The degree of government intrusion enacted through the ACA is difficult to over-emphasize. It structurally affects the length of time that doctors can spend with patients, threatens doctor-patient confidentiality, and even affects the content of what doctors can ask about or discuss regardless of the relevance to the patient's condition. [30]

For physicians and their patients, perhaps the worse provisions of the ACA are hidden by a lack of transparency, and their effects remain unknown today. However, it seems sure that "The government will now be calling the shots," [30] and all of our foundational principles will be upended by the new healthcare law. An essential tenet of patient empowerment must be for patients and all stakeholders to demand of our government, the right to practice those principles.

IMPACT OF MEDICAID EXPANSION ON CONSUMER ACCESS, QUALITY OF CARE, AND INCREASING COSTS

According to the Congressional Budget Office, the ACA will force 17 million Americans into Medicaid, in what the WHO has called the developed world's 37th worst health care system. [32][33]

Medicaid was originally intended as a safety net for the poor, and not as a large-scale health insurance plan. Simply expanding the numbers of patients assigned Medicaid cards, is not the same thing as expanding actual access to healthcare. In fact, as stated by the Kaiser Family Foundation, an organization that is generally favorable to the ACA: "...added demand in numbers of patients, without a concomitant re-scaling of the system will worsen patient dissatisfaction as individuals face longer wait times, increased costs, and new frustrations caused by the accompanying decrease in the quality of care." [34]

In his book, "How Medicaid Fails the Poor," Avik Roy, senior fellow at the Manhattan Institute illustrates how Medicaid, rather than being helpful, is distinctly harmful to low-income Americans who are already struggling. Medicaid has never risen to the level of value that would allow low income patients gain access to mainstream healthcare "as neither the federal government nor the states were willing to spend the money that would have been required" according to Roy. Study after study shows that patients on Medicaid do no better, and often worse, than those with no insurance at all. [35]

Roy calls that "the massive fallacy at the heart of Medicaid, and therefore at the heart of Obamacare," the idea that health insurance equals healthcare. Patients on Medicare who were undergoing surgery were 45 percent more likely to die before leaving the hospital than those with private insurance; the uninsured were 74 percent more likely; and Medicaid patients were 93 percent more likely. That is to say, "despite the fact that we will soon spend more than $500 billion a year on Medicaid, Medicaid beneficiaries, on average, fared slightly worse than those with no insurance at all." [35]

This argument, that Medicaid was not making poor people healthier, is so important, yet seems so counterintuitive, especially to those who believe in the efficacy of government programs, that it is necessary to demonstrate how this point has been proven by two of the most powerful and well-regarded studies in the health insurance arena. To understand these studies is to prove facts that most progressives dismiss entirely.

In the most important health insurance study ever conducted, researchers at the RAND Corporation devised an experiment that has ongoing ramifications for healthcare reform. In that study, two key questions were asked: how much more medical care will people use if it is provided free of charge, and what are the consequences for their health? Taking steps to experimentally equalize factors for urban and rural populations, participants were enrolled in a range of insurance plans requiring different levels of co-payment for medical care, from zero to 95 percent. The result was that in plans that reimbursed a higher proportion of the bill, patients used substantially more services and regardless of the amount of services, the effect on the health of the average person was negligible. [36][37][38][39]

Now that it has been shown that the amount of insurance one has seems to have little or no effect on the health of the average person, one might ask whether having health insurance at all make people healthier?[38] A central tenet of the ACA is that its expansion of Medicaid to cover the uninsured would save thousands of lives a year. The idea that some insurance coverage would be better than none had not been challenged. Now, a study out of Oregon casts further doubt on the fundamental premise that insurance improves health outcomes.

In 2008, an infrequent, ready-made experiment presented itself to the people of Oregon. The state government had enough money to extend its' Medicaid program by 10,000 low-income people. However, many more were eligible. A randomized, state lottery was set-up to determine who would get coverage, and to compare the health outcomes of about 6,000 people who won the lottery. An additional, equal sized group of lottery 'losers' was used as controls. Thus emerged one of the best circumstances in which to test the effects of public policies. [38]

The Oregon Health Study, published in May, 2013 in the New England Journal of Medicine, found much the same thing that the RAND Health Insurance. The experiment had shown, namely, that Medicaid coverage generated no significant improvements in measured physical health outcomes in the first 2 years. There were some benefits from having the insurance, to be sure, [38] and no one is advocating eliminating health insurance for anyone. But, there is a better, cheaper, safer way of providing access to healthcare for everyone than the ACA provides.[35][38]

Both the RAND study and the Oregon study undermine the case for the vast expansion of Medicaid provided in the ACA. "Most U.S. health insurance today, thanks to the tax preference for employer-provided insurance, is not real insurance at all. Real insurance should pay for rare, expensive, and unwelcome events, such as your house's burning down. It doesn't make sense to insure for routine expenses, like repainting your living room. The Oregon Health Study suggests that insurance isn't necessary for people to get what are now, for people of a certain age, routine items such as blood-pressure medicine.[38] Maybe government should help poor people pay for routine items and procedures directly. Blood sugar, blood pressure, and cholesterol levels can be treated with relatively inexpensive generic drugs. Medicaid coverage may result in more people getting heart-bypass surgery and needing expensive drugs for rare ailments. But that is another way of saying that health insurance as we know it may not do much to improve the treatment of common health problems. Americans have come to expect health insurance to pay for routine treatments. Obamacare reinforces that in its requirements for coverage and makes it more difficult for many to insure against catastrophic health-care expenses. [35][38]

Virtually every serious study of consumer-directed healthcare has reached conclusions similar to the original RAND research. And in addition, a second conclusion set the stage to place the freedoms squarely back with the consumers: that people with high-deductible plans and HSAs spend about 30 percent less on healthcare than those with conventional coverage, with no apparent adverse effects on health. [38]

The RAND HIE and Oregon Insurance Study prove, according to Avik Roy, [35] that the exorbitant cost of covering the uninsured with Medicaid does not make patients healthier. Balance that with the proposition that there are several, well studied market-based alternatives to Medicaid that would offer uninsured, low-income Americans the opportunity to see the doctor of their choice and gain access to high quality, private-sector health care.

Most of these strategies involve giving uncovered patients a combination of Health Savings Accounts, which can empower all patients of any income level (on a sliding scale based upon income) to pay for many routine medical services with cash rather than inappropriately with health insurance which is not meant as a pre-payment system for all healthcare expenses. Health insurance should be reserved for catastrophic, potentially bankrupting events. That is precisely what affordable, high deductible health insurance was made to do. This strategy is far from hypothetical. For example, when in Indiana, patients on Medicaid were also given an inexpensive combination of high deductible insurance and subsidized health-savings accounts, the program enjoyed a 98 percent approval. However, the Obama administration has declined to renew Indiana's waiver to continue this program, insisting that it be replaced by traditional Medicaid. [37]

Bold thinkers such as John C Goodman, the father of Health Savings Accounts (HSA), and healthcare analyst, Avik Roy, have put forward their versions of health insurance strategies that could replace the need for Medicaid, at significant savings, and could be implemented immediately.

Roy gives an expanded plan that would guarantee low-income consumers the standard of care that seems prohibitive by the ACA. He says: "But let's not tinker around the edges with Medicaid...Let's build from scratch a new health program for low-income Americans, one that would actually offer better health care than many wealthy Americans receive." [35][37]

Roy suggests paying a primary-care physician $80 a month to see each patient, whether he is healthy or sick". Low-income patients would have their own concierge physicians, who would be contracted to see their paying patients without concern or delay. Additional fees for service, charges for other family members, and subsidized, high-deductible insurance against catastrophic events could be paid out of the HSA's subsidies. [35]

Taking this thinking one step further, this strategy could become a workable model for every American. Only the presence or absence and level of subsidies would vary, and more services could be added to the insurance plan as consumers who could pay more, demand it. And, the savings of eliminating Medicaid would be staggering. [35]

REFERENCES

1. Top 10 Takeaways: Public Opinion on the Affordable Care Act Http://www.aei.org/publication/top-10-takeaways-public-opinion-on-the-affordable-care-act/

2. Gallup: Obamacare popularity in free fall, reaches lowest rating in poll's history, http://hotair.com/archives/2014/11/17/gallup-obamacare-popularity-in-free-fall-reaches-lowest-rating-in-polls-history/

3. Public Approval of Health Care Law, http://www.realclearpolitics.com/epolls/other/obama_and_democrats_health_care_plan-1130.htm

4. http://www.washingtontimes.com/news/2014/oct/28/obamacare-sends-health-premiums-skyrocketing-by-as/?page=all

5. Health Plan Premiums Are Skyrocketing According To New Survey Of 148 Insurance Brokers, With Delaware Up 100%, California 53%, Florida 37%, Pennsylvania 28% Scott Gottlieb http://www.forbes.com/sites/scottgottlieb/2014/04/07/health-plan-premiums-are-skyrocketing-according-to-new-survey-of-148-insurance-brokers-analysts-blame-obamacare/

6. http://www.aetna.com/health-reform-connection/aetnas-vision/facts-about-costs.html

7. http://www.ahip.org/Issues/Rising-Health-Care-Costs.aspx

8. (http://www.newsmax.com/Newsmax-Tv/rand-paul-obama-govern-

ment-socialism/2014/02/05/id/551134/)

9. http://www.independentsentinel.com/rand-paul-the-united-states-is-being-turned-into-a-socialist-nightmare/

10. http://thedailyshow.cc.com/videos/xh6isx/exclusive---charles-krauthammer-extended-interview-pt-1, 2, 3.

11. Atlas, S.W., Traitel, J. & Fellow, S., 2014. Scott W. Atlas Website.

12. http://hotair.com/archives/2009/08/04/obama-2003-uncut-sure-i-support-single-payer-health-care/

13. http://healthblog.ncpa.org/the-collectivist-mind/#sthash.MRJTQXIu.dpuf trust collective action more than they trust individual action.

14. http://healthblog.ncpa.org/the-collectivist-mind/#sthash.MRJTQXIu.dpuf ., 2009.

15. Marxist Equality. (July). http://www.rightsidenews.com/2009072319138/editorial/us-opinion-and-editorial/marxist-equality.html and Cherry, B.R.R., The Judeo-Christian Values of America. http://www.americanthinker.com/2007/09/the_judeochristian_values_of_a.html

16. Real Clear Markets - The Government Can't Control Health Care Costs realclearmarkets.com · by Matt Kibbe · August 25, 2009 https://www.instapaper.com/read/513056236

17. Three Reasons Why Government Can't Run Health Care | Human Events humanevents.com · August 26, 2009 https://www.instapaper.com/read/488927197

18. "A fatal wait: Veterans languish and die on a VA hospital's secret list," Scott Bronstein and Drew Griffin, CNN Investigations updated 9:19 PM EDT, Wed April 23, 2014, http://www.cnn.com/2014/04/23/health/veterans-dying-health-care-delays/

19. How Medicaid Fails the Poor (Encounter Broadsides) Paperback – November 12, 2013 by Avik Roy (Author)

20. http://www.americanthinker.com/articles/2013/12/the_future_of_medical_specialists_under_the_affordable_care_act.html

21. Articles: The Future of Medical Specialists under the Affordable Care Act americanthinker.com· December 11, 2013

22. 5 ways the Affordable Care Act will transform primary care practices medical economics. modern medicine.com · by Debra Beaulieu· Decem-

ber 25, 2013

23. Obamacare's Impact on Doctors—An Update heritage.org· by Alyene Senger· August 23, 2013

24. Betsy McCaughey book, Obamacare's Impact on Doctors—An Update heritage.org · by Alyene Senger · August 23, 2013.

25. How The Affordable Care Act Will Affect Doctors | The Health Care Blog thehealthcareblog.com· by Tevi Troy· June 15, 2012

26. Nearly 1/4 of doctors may opt out of Obamacare exchanges in 2015 - Hot Air

27. Senate: Insurers Should Cover Mammos for 40-Year-Olds- Note: This had to be reversed because of the clamor it caused by women. But examples like this are destined to take place, and the ACAs regulators won't give-in so easily next time.

28. AAOS, Physician Patient Communication. Importance of Good Communication in the Physician-Patient Relationship Information Statement - AAOS

29. http://www.beckershospitalreview.com/hospital-physician-relationships/survey-physician-patient-relationship-more-important-than-treatment-in-patient-satisfaction.html

30. The Impact of the Affordable Care Act on the Health Care Workforce

31. William Osler: A Life in Medicine-Michael Bliss, Note: "Listen to your patient, he is telling you the diagnosis," teaches William Osler.

32. WHO.org 2000 Health Systems: Improving Performance.

33. Scott W Atlas, 2011. The Worst Study Ever ? , (April). The Worst Study Ever? - Commentary Magazine

34. Why 31 million people will remain uninsured under ObamaCare

35. How Medicaid Fails the Poor (Encounter Broadsides) by Avik Roy Kindle edition loc. 17.

36. Free for All? Lessons from the RAND Health Insurance Experiment, Joseph P. Newhouse, Insurance Experiment Group

37. http://www.rand.org/pubs/commercial_books/CB199.html Harvard University Press, 1993 in Goodman, John C. (2012-06-01).

38. Does having health insurance make people healthier Barone, M., 2013. Washington Examiner

39. Uncontrolled: The Surprising Payoff of Trial-and-Error for Business, Politics, and Society, Manzi, Jim in Goodman, John C. (2012-06-01).

*   (http://www.galen.org/medicaid-expansion-and-obamacare/)

**   (http://www.forbes.com/sites/theapothecary/2013/05/02/oregon-study-medicaid-had-no-significant-effect-on-health-outcomes-vs-being-uninsured/)

CHAPTER EIGHT:

FIRST PRINCIPLES AND THE ROLE OF BIG GOVERNMENT IN U.S. HEALTHCARE REFORM

Central to building exceptionalism into healthcare is an understanding of the relationship between America's first principles and our healthcare system. First principles, as stated in the Declaration of Independence and the Constitution include limited government -- where the government can only do what the people give it the power to do, makes the individual sovereign and not the state, and equality means equality under the law, not the "equal" redistribution of wealth. Under the constitution, individuals have the right to control their personal property. It is a moral imperative, not legal, that drives the American character to be charitable, and provide healthcare to our fellow man who is incapable of providing for himself.

These values gave rise to American exceptionalism when the country was founded, and a century later to American medical exceptionalism. These principles also form the basis for the role of government in U.S. healthcare reform. [1]

THE INFLUENCE OF THE PROGRESSIVE WORLDVIEW ON U.S. HEALTHCARE REFORM

A generation before Franklin Roosevelt's New Deal, "American politics and intellectual culture were dominated by America's original big government liberals, the Progressives, who sought a thorough transformation in America's principles of government, from one permanently dedicated to securing individual liberty to one that had progressed to take on any and all social and economic ills." according to R.J. Pestritto, Shipley Professor of the American Constitution at Hillsdale College. [2][3][4] Early Progressives openly denounced the sources of America's first principles, the Declaration of Independence and US. Constitution. Perhaps limited government more suited a country that had just come through a revolutionary war against a despotic king George III, they argued. Progressives saw the early 20th century as a time to move on from the Founders' principles.

Long before Barrack Obama, Woodrow Wilson believed that "the original intention of the separation of powers system could be circumvented, and the enhanced presidency could be a means energizing the kind of active national government that the progressive agenda required." [2][3][4] Wilson, for example, once warned that "if you want to understand the real Declaration of Independence, do not repeat the preface."[4] Theodore Roosevelt, when using the federal government to take over private businesses during the 1902 coal strike, is reported to have remarked, "To hell with the Constitution when people want coal!" [2][3][4]

Progressives have continued to press for ideas that we fought wars to prevent. Each subsequent Democrat president has attempted to expand government and the role of the presidency as means of negating those principles. The ACA, however, is their greatest triumph.

In his book, "Replacing Obamacare: The Cato Institute on Health Care Reform," Michael Tanner says: "The healthcare law that President Barack Obama signed in March, 2010 stands among the most sweeping pieces of social legislation in United States history." By 2014, he says, "it will have conscripted nearly the entire U.S. population into a compulsory health insurance scheme, with tentacles reaching out to all quadrants of healthcare delivery, financing, and regulation."[5]

Like the original Progressives, Wilson, Theodore Roosevelt and others, [2][3][4] President Obama maintains that only the federal government can adequately address a nation's healthcare needs, matching the massive and complex problem with an equally massive and complex solution. Advocates maintain that government – "with its size, infrastructure, and power" – is best equipped to deliver such a solution on a national scale through a "single-payer" model, where one entity— the central government—"collects all health care fees and pays all health care-related costs, and therefore makes every decision regarding every stakeholder in the healthcare system". [4]

Others of his ilk, the architects of the ACA, likewise believe that in order to have complete control, government needs to dismantle and replace the existing system rather than improve upon a century of excellence. It is not surprising that they see our entire healthcare system as an embarrassment and in need of being replaced:

"The American healthcare system is a dysfunctional mess." So opens his book, "Healthcare Guaranteed: A Simple, Secure Solution for America," the alternative healthcare plan by Ezekiel Emanuel MD. PhD, a plan that was destined to become the ACA. [6]

Emanuel, one of the chief architects of the ACA, and a close Obama aide, blames the dysfunction on everyone, except Big Government. "Everyone involved in the healthcare system is in some way at fault." He says that healthcare corporations are guilty of fraud, pharmaceutical companies prey on desperate patients, and physicians routinely perform unnecessary operations. And, what about the $2.8 trillion that the government expends on our "sickly" system, the "skimpy" and "lacking" health insurance, absence of preventative care and screening, and poor performance in clinically caring for patients with heart attacks or pneumonia? He does mention "flawed policies" but forgets to attribute them to the big-government lawmakers who enacted those policies. [6] When faced with mounting government control, one need merely ask, "Is more of the same government that brought us these results going to make things better? Or, what large system has government bureaucracies ever managed efficiently?"

Emanuel makes these points: "the major shortcomings of American healthcare are the result of deep and irreparable flaws in the way the country finances, organizes, and delivers care." [6] Emanuel and others are deluded by their political worldview if they think that more government can repair those flaws by unilaterally imposing more than 21 new or higher taxes* on American families and small businesses.[7] and an Independent Payment Advisory Board (IPAB) which, outside of the influence of political processes and pressures, has the power to force arbitrary across-the-board cuts to physicians and other providers, or ration Medicare services. [8] The ACA also gives Government complete control over doctor decisions, and forms 59 new boards and agencies to regulate all aspects of the healthcare system. [9]

Government-controlled medicine requires doctors, hospitals and other providers to follow overly restrictive regulations. Government determines what services are provided, the appropriate and recommended treatment, when and where you can get that treatment, and what fees doctors are paid. [10] Other countries that have instituted such systems are now beginning to understand their futility and are instituting free market healthcare such as the UK.

The two fundamental flaws in government-controlled healthcare are its immorality and inefficacy. The government treats doctors, hospitals and patients as "widgets and diminish, if not eliminate, the ability, responsibility, and power that individuals have to manage their own health care."[10] Under these plans, individuals have little power or choice over their provider, treatment or payment. Someone else, such as a bureaucrat, with little or no accountability, makes those decisions for every doctor, hospital, insurer, and patient.[10] Furthermore, government is incapable of formulating and carrying out sustainable, constructive strategies that would lead to good healthcare systems, as I demonstrate in this book.

Emanuel correctly states that the system's "nearly 1 million acute hospital beds, 850,000 physicians, 2.5 million nurses, about 1,000 health insurance companies, and more than 3 billion prescriptions....make it so difficult to accurately predict how any proposed change will affect... stakeholders, much less individual families." Yet his book, and later the ACA, itself, proposes innumerable changes without the ability to accurately predict their effects through untested, even as yet unwritten, pilot projects, despite the fact that his anti-constitutional worldview has been in the minority among the American people before and after the ACA was passed. [11]

One of the best indications that the ACA is destined for failure was Vermont's decision at the end of 2014 to abandon the state's ambitious plans to build a single-payer, universal healthcare system, because it would result in massive tax hikes according to its' Governor, Peter Shumlin (D). It would cause excessive "economic disruption and risks" to small businesses and individual citizens.[12]

GOVERNMENT INTRUSION ON FIRST PRINCIPLES IN HEALTHCARE REFORM

The Founders of the American Republic understood that the potential for government to consolidate its power was the greatest single threat to liberty, according to Robert Moffit, PhD, senior fellow in The Heritage Foundation's Center for Health Policy Studies. [13] The evidence from government-run healthcare systems around the world is exceedingly clear. As Cato Institute senior fellow, Michael Tanner, [26] puts it: "In countries weighted heavily toward government control, people are most likely to face waiting lists, rationing, restrictions on physician choice, and other obstacles to care." By contrast," other healthcare systems are "successful to the degree that they incorporate market mechanisms such as competition, cost-consciousness, market prices, and consumer choice, and eschew centralized government control."[14]

The Progressive movement advocates big government as the best means to attain societal ends. However, many historians and politicians believe that big government is a cover for elites to grab power by always promising a form of utopia. History bears out that those governments always fail, and there are always elites attempting to run the government. [28] We now know that the "fundamental transformation of government" that President Barack Obama surreptitiously engineered within the ACA was such a form of government.

Our government does not need to be transformed. We need to re-dedicate ourselves to first principles. We must look to President Ronald Reagan who said: "Government is not a solution to our problem, government is the problem." [16] As we will see, increasing intrusion by government has led to the real world proof of government's inability to fix healthcare's weaknesses.

Unlike the previous historical experiments whose principles rested with exceptionalism, the ACA was designed to cut back on most of the valuable assets of U.S. healthcare by reducing overall excellence in order to achieve 'forced equality of outcome.'

CAN THE ROLE OF GOVERNMENT BE CHANGED UNDER THE ACA?

We have a first principle obligation to exercise our right to limit government to work for us, and take action when it works against our will. Obviously, the most important action would be to vote for an advocate of repeal in the next Presidential election.

As long as the ACA remains intact and functional, no fundamental changes in its intrusive provisions are likely. Some changes can be made at the margins without repeal of the law assuming the sitting President is willing to sign the new reform measures into law. President Obama seems unlikely to be a willing partner with the Republican majority in both houses of Congress, thereby delaying change until the 2016 election. Regardless of the party affiliation of the next President, some steps can be taken if repeal, for whatever reason, is taken off the table. In the event that President Obama is willing to work with the Republican majorities in both houses of Congress, there are some changes that can be taken without repealing the law, that would partially restore some first principle intent. Otherwise, the Congress should consider passing purely symbolic bills, knowing that they would be vetoed by the President.

In my view, Congress must go on record as favoring complete repeal of the ACA. The legislative machinations of repeal have been reported by some experts as daunting. Its tentacles are extensive, and, if legislators must repeal incrementally, it is important that this process be initiated as soon as possible. In addition, there must be a highly acceptable alternative plan waiting in the wings, ready for immediate enactment when the ACA is repealed.[20] The law should be openly rebuked lest vestiges be tacitly perceived as agreeable to Republicans. Republicans are requesting that an alternative bill be written before they commit to repeal ACA.

The fact that some steps to modify the ACA could be taken if complete repeal proves impossible is born out by the fact that at least 46 changes have been made to the law after its enactment. President Obama has made 28 unilateral changes to the law by

Executive orders or memoranda, something some experts believe were performed extra-constitutionally. [18]

Moreover, in January, 2015 the House of Representatives quickly took up changes to the ACA that could result in the beginning of dismantling the law. They changed the definition of a full-time work week to 40 hours. The longer workweek definition would mean fewer workers must be offered health insurance by their employer under the health law's employer mandate. The House has cleared more than 50 assorted measures to repeal or roll back Obamacare that it could send on to the GOP-controlled Senate, potentially forcing President Barack Obama to either accept changes to his signature domestic achievement or use his veto power. [30]

REFERENCES

1. Uhlmann, Eric Luis, American Moral Exceptionalism

2. American Progressivism, R.J. Pestritto,Shipley Professor of the American Constitution at Hillsdale College, glennbeck.com · April 16, 2009

3. http://www.glennbeck.com/content/articles/article/198/23936 /

4. http://www.discoverthenetworks.org/guideDesc.asp?catid=93&type=issue

5. Tanner, Michael D.; Cannon, Michael F. (2012-07-25). Replacing Obamacare: The Cato Institute on Health Care Reform (Kindle Locations 4731-4733). Cato Institute. Kindle Edition.

6. Emanuel, Ezekiel (2009-02-23). Healthcare, Guaranteed: A Simple, Secure Solution for America (p. 1). Public Affairs. Kindle Edition.

7. Full List of Obamacare Tax Hikes: Listed by Size of Tax Hike atr.org, June 29, 2012

8. http://www.ama-assn.org/ama/pub/advocacy/topics/independent-payment-advisory-board.page

9. http://www.nationalreview.com/critical-condition/304361/top-ten-worst-things-obamacare-grace-marie-turner

10. Freedom and Individual Rights in Medicine westandfirm.org http://www.westandfirm.org/

11. Liberal Self-Identification Edges Up to New High in 2013

12. http://humanevents.com/2014/12/18/single-payer-health-care-dies-in-vermont/

13. Moffit http://www.heritage.org/research/lecture/2011/04/reforming-health-care-on-the-foundation-of-first-principles

14. The Grass Is Not Always Greener A Look at National Health Care Systems Around the World by Michael Tanner

15. Why Socialism Failed, Collectivism Is Based on Faulty Principles JUNE 01, 1995 by Mark Perry.

16. http://fee.org/the_freeman/detail/why-socialism-failed First Inaugural Address, January 20, 1981

17. Capretta, How to Replace Obamacare > Publications > National Affairs

18. 46 Changes to Obamacare...So Far. January 7, 2015, By Tyler Hartsfield and Grace-Marie Turner http://www.galen.org/newsletters/changes-to-obamacare-so-far/

19. http://www.politico.com/story/2015/01/obamacare-repeal-house-work-week-114089.html#ixzz3OjWR4F1s

20. http://www.nationalaffairs.com/publications/detail/how-to-replace-obamacare

* http://www.washingtonpost.com/blogs/fact-checker/post/how-many-pages-of-regulations-for-obamacare/2013/05/14/61eec914-bcf9-11e2-9b09-1638acc3942e_blog.html

CHAPTER NINE:

FIRST PRINCIPLES AND THE ROLE OF THE FREE MARKET IN U.S. HEALTHCARE REFORM

THE AMERICAN CHARACTER

The Founding Fathers realized that all political systems were fragile,[1] and we know that goes for healthcare as well. However, they left a legacy to guide us.

Representative Paul Ryan, Chairman of the House Budget Committee, and Republican Vice-Presidential nominee in 2012, addressed the issue of the American character, and its effect on healthcare reform.[2] Representative Ryan reminds us that government's mission was limited to creating conditions where men and women can achieve their potential. This means, in part, taking responsibility for their own lives, and to pursue happiness through "charity, self-restraint, industriousness, enterprise creativity, and hard work, and not through victimization, or passive handouts." [2]

Americans also expect their healthcare to be allowed to continue, grow, and improve without undue government intrusion. The economist, Robert Nozick, famously argued, that a just society is one where government's only legitimate function was to enforce contracts, and protect citizens against violence, theft and fraud, resulting in an unfettered free market.[3]

Instead, Obamacare has betrayed these values, putting us in danger of total government control, where the free market is anathema to his worldview. The ACA has removed any chance that healthcare can be reformed based upon American values. A stroke of his pen negated many of the American values that made our healthcare system exceptional.

The ACA imposes a quasi-collectivist system, devoid of deference to our uniquely American values. Progressives have taken advantage of a manufactured healthcare crisis to promote and expand their goal of collectivism, robbing us of our American values of freedom, individualism, and right of property. "And, no right to property is more important than one's ownership of his own body. [4]

FREE MARKETS AND AMERICAN EXCEPTIONALISM

Progressives see the economy as a zero sum game, where, as the affluent become richer and get a bigger piece of the pie, there is less for low-income citizens who must settle for smaller and smaller pieces. However, the economy is not a zero sum game simply because economies expand. The pie gets bigger. As it does, everyone has an opportunity in place to earn a bigger piece of the pie. With their worldview imposed, such opportunities are hidden in order for Progressives to maintain control, stifle economic growth, and redistribute money. Trying to force material equality depletes creativity and with it, any chance for exceptionalism. Rather than waiting for handouts of redistributed money, those who assume the responsibility to work hard to succeed in society are often rewarded with the mobility to improve their economic condition, a characteristic that only exists as a result of American exceptionalism.

Simply put, a free market is a form of economy that allows forces of supply and demand to regulate prices, unfettered by government regulation, leading to a just society.[3] In such an economy, when one's own property results in financial gain, instead of causing an equivalent loss to another, it leads to improvements in the general economy to the benefit of all participants. This is free market capitalism, the most morally just model of economy, which "has done more to empower people and raise living standards than any other force in history."[5] "Everywhere that capitalism subsequently has taken hold, national wealth increases and poverty falls. And where capitalism has not allowed to take hold, people remain impoverished.[6]

That simple set of facts form the basis for free market capitalism; why it is morally just to propagate it, and immoral to substitute collectivism in its place.

THE MYTH THAT AMERICAN HEALTHCARE HAS FAILED IN THE FREE MARKET

It is argued by opponents of U.S. Healthcare, that our system has had its chance in the free market, and failed.[7] However, advocates point out that U.S. healthcare has never existed in a free market. The U.S. market has always been characterized by distortions resulting from "overly restrictive policies, Medicare, Medicaid, and tax subsidies...[with] federal policies primarily responsible for driving up costs and making health insurance unaffordable for so many Americans."[8] says Kevin D. Dayaratna, Ph.D. of the Heritage Foundation. He goes on, "It is therefore incorrect to look at the broad performance of the largely uncompetitive American healthcare system and make judgments about whether a competitive health system would work well or not."

In order for healthcare to thrive in a laissez-faire free market as prescribed by first principles, certain reforms are necessary to remove those distortions, and level the playing field.

REFORM MEASURES: A CONSUMER-CENTERED HEALTHCARE MODEL IN THE FREE MARKET

The first objective of fashioning our healthcare system for entry into a free market is to recognize that a free-market economy is not a zero sum game, a fixed size that must be divvied-up by everyone. When the reforms that I mention are implemented, the distorted forces of healthcare's third parties will be replaced by a more efficient, less-costly, and more flexible environment. Second, we must toss-off the incorrect notion that there are only two ways of reforming healthcare, one, to our status quo prior to 2010, and the other by adhering to the ACA, both being failures in their own way. There are good alternatives. Our legacy, from the Founding Fathers of America, and from the Founders of American Medicine in Baltimore, provides a road map to exceptionalism. In addition, we must bear in mind, as I have discussed throughout this book, governments are incapable of creating and sustaining workable healthcare systems.

Fortunately, in today's skeptical age, an enormous amount of research and thought have generated compelling evidence for the benefits of market-driven healthcare systems. [8][9][10]

CHOICE OF HEALTHCARE PLANS SHOULD BE IN THE HANDS OF THE CONSUMER.

Heritage Foundation senior fellow, Robert Moffit explains that "In a free-market system, consumers would have the ability to choose how to meet their health insurance needs, taxpayers would benefit from a more efficient and affordable system, and above all, patients, with their doctors, should make their own health care decisions free from government interference." [11]

Mandates would be excluded, and tax breaks would be evened-out between employees who receive their health insurance from employers as "fringe benefits," versus those purchasing individual health plans who are forced to pay with their own after-tax dollars.

Americans would not only choose the plans that best suit their needs and the needs of their families; they would own their insurance, unrelated to employment or geographical location. The insured would then be able to purchase insurance policies that "they can take with them from job to job' (portability) [12] says James Capretta, former associate director at the White House's Office of Management and Budget, and Senior Fellow at the Ethics and Public Policy Center, at the American Enterprise Institute.

No one would be denied health insurance, even those with pre-existing conditions. Of course, such policies will be more costly than for consumers who are well. Allowing the cost to respond to the natural market forces by increasing keeps overall health insurance more balanced with fewer perverse incentives. Higher government subsidies will be require to enable low-income consumers to afford these policies, to be sure. Since passage of the ACA, far fewer applicants with pre-existing conditions have applied. [12] In fact, as reported in the Federal Register [15] the government has ended the Pre-Existing Condition Insurance Plan (PCIP) of the ACA because the program's overall costs became too extreme because many of the patients had higher-than-anticipated medical bills, despite the relatively low enrollment. [14] This does not bode well for ACA exchanges also, and may be a reason why employer mandated exchanges were delayed. [15]

HEALTH SAVINGS ACCOUNT (HSA) AND HIGH DEDUCTIBLE LOW COST (HDLC) CATASTROPHE INSURANCE

Congress should reform the tax treatment of healthcare by enlarging health savings accounts that were lowered by the ACA. A tax-free health savings account (HSA) should be offered together with a policy that has a higher deductible, but offers protection in the event of a catastrophic illness. As one of several new consumer-driven health options, HSAs encourage patients to take control of their own healthcare, providing financial incentives for consumers to serve as wise healthcare purchasers with protection against bankruptcy if medical bills become prohibitive when catastrophic illnesses occur.

Congress should reform Medicare and Medicaid to gradually transition to fiscally responsible programs which would support individuals in need, and give them the same consumer choices and market controls available to Americans who purchase their own health insurance.

REFORM OF HEALTHCARE DELIVERY

What the U.S. Healthcare system needs is radical innovation, not radical reform.

Following the precepts of our first principles will have a profound effect on healthcare delivery reform. We will re-gain the freedoms to ethically pursue the doctor-patient relationship in confidence, to provide innovations that will preserve our prior availability of bio-technical, diagnostic and therapeutic devices, and to allow the free market to determine doctors fees and make other costs more transparent. These steps will help to preserve one of our great birthrights, the availability of a sufficient number of expert physician specialists, all available without the need to ration care through excessive waiting.

But, this is just a beginning. Critics of our excellent healthcare system have brought to light serious problems that must be addressed going forward. In addition to cost, access and safety which will be positively impacted by embracing first principles once again, there are additional scientific and bioethical problems that will take many years to control, including:

Fragmentation of care Inherent in the vastness of any

healthcare system are problems that arise when individuals, groups or organizations strive to achieve autonomy, while at the same time requiring interoperability. Will reformers take the same approach as architects of the ACA by trying to reduce the problem through intrusive laws that run contrary to first principles? Or, will multiple islands of excellence arise, locally and regionally, close to the people they intend to help, each their own experimental pilot projects, with the potential to point the way toward future solutions?

Is healthcare still a growth industry? Can we transform the enormous increase in the workforce that will arise from proper healthcare reform into a growth sector that positively impacts upon our economy?

Bio-medical research Has there been, as some experts believe, a halt in the progress of bio-medical research, and can it be blamed the bio-medical model largely developed by the Hopkins group? Or, do answers to this question lie within normal translational hurdles that would require changes in how time and budget are allocated for research? And how would such changes impact "pure research" that has historically been so fruitful?

Game changing technologies What will be the effects of game-changing technologies such as genomic medicine on the current clinical paradigm? And, how will those challenges be met bio-ethically?

We, perhaps, should make it part of our national will to call for a 21st Century healthcare reform project similar to the moon missions in the 1960's. Unlike the slapdash approach of the ACA, viable healthcare reform will take a generation or more to come within grips of these and the many additional problems that face our system. How we organize and go forward with that national enterprise will impact on its success. We must have a zero tolerance for failure.

HEALTHCARE REFORM AND ECONOMIC FREEDOM

In their book, "Freedom Manifesto: Why Free Markets Are Moral and Big Government Isn't," [16] authors Steve Forbes and Elizabeth Ames ask the central question of our time: "Are we a country founded on the values of freedom and limited government, as envisioned by the founding fathers in the Declaration of Independence and the Constitution? Or, do we want to become a European-style socialist democracy?" Their answer was rooted in pragmatism, that the system that worked best for the public good today is the correct one.

The answer to that question is also the central theme of this book. I have attempted to describe why the U.S. healthcare system prior to passage of the ACA was exceptional, not only because of its inherent morality, derived from America's first principles, and its scientific excellence, derived from medical leaders such as those in the Hopkins experiment, but also because it out-performs collectivist systems, and is overwhelmingly preferred by Americans. In order to address its weaknesses we must also transform our healthcare system, not into the constrained, oppressed system that would result from the ACA, but through economic freedom, into a growth industry in a vigorous, free market environment.

Restoring American medical exceptionalism means we must re-dedicate ourselves to those same, fragile principles that make up our American values. We must once again take our place in what Sir William Osler called our common medical lineage, and once again bring forward relevant lessons from history through to patient-centered and personalized healthcare models of today, while pursuing game-changing technological innovations such as digital and genomic medicine, and being open to those we have yet to imagine. In return, dazzling scientific achievements and incomparable healthcare are waiting to be re-born through modern healthcare reform.

REFERENCE

1   Murray, Charles (2013-07-05). American Exceptionalism: An Experiment in History (Values and Capitalism) (Kindle Locations 392-397). Aei Press. Kindle Edition.

2   spectator.org, July 23, 2009 .http://spectator.org/articles/41203/ health-care-reform-and-american-character (Health Care Reform and the American Character, Rep. Paul Ryan.)

3. Why Nozick Matters, http://mises.org/library/why-nozick-matters

4. Ralston, R.E., 2013. American Health Care : Essential Principles and 50 Common Fallacies

5. Capitalism's Triumph: Occupy Wall Street is wrong — it's the best system for everyone. By Michael Tanner, SEPTEMBER 18, 2013http://www. nationalreview.com/article/358771/capitalisms-triumph-michael-tanner

6. Why Capitalism Has an Image Problem By CHARLES MURRAY Updated July 30, 2012, The Wall Street Journal Online

7. The Myth of 'Market Failure' in Health Care OCTOBER 30, 2009 http:// www.cato.org/blog/myth-market-failure-health-care.)

8. Compelling Evidence Makes the Case for a Market-Driven Health Care System heritage.org · by Kevin D. Dayaratna, Ph.D. December 20, 2013

9. (Yes, Mr. President, A Free Market Can Fix Health , Policy Analysis, Cannon, M.F., 1996. Cato Institute)

10. The 2014 Physician's Prescription for Healthcare Reform docs4patient-care.org, http://www.docs4patientcare.org/prescription)

11. Moffit and Roberts, J.M. & Olson, R., How Economic Freedom Promotes Better Health Care, Education, and Environmental Quality.

12. After Repeal of Obamacare: Moving to Patient-Centered, Market-Based Health Care

13. (https://www.federalregister.gov/articles/2013/05/22/2013-12145/pre-existing-condition-insurance-plan-program)

14. (https://www.bcbsm.com/health-care-reform/reform-alerts/pre-existing-condition-ins-plan-announces-closure-to-new-enrollment.html)

15. (http://www.forbes.com/sites/gracemarieturner/2013/04/10/a-temporaray-insurance-program-foretells-exploding-obamacare-costs/)

16. Freedom Manifesto: Why Free Markets Are Moral and Big Government Isn't," authors Steve Forbes and Elizabeth Ames

INDEX

ABOUT THE AUTHOR

DR. MYLES SAUNDERS is a Diplomat of the American Board of Neurological Surgery. Since 1998, Dr. Saunders has worked full time in the eHealth Industry, primarily in the areas of telemedicine, tele-radiology and medical informatics. As a corporate advisor, he has worked closely with such companies as IdeaLab, Inc. (Pasadena, California), and Odell International (Charlotte, North Carolina) developing a wide range of online medical products and services. As Founder and Chairman of HealthAddress, Inc., he has collaborated to bring telemedicine and teleradiology services to domestic and offshore clients. Dr. Saunders has been advisor in eHealth to HH Sheikh Mohammed bin Rashid al Maktoum, leader of the Emirate of Dubai, and Vice-President of the United Arab Emirates as well as multiple business and scientific leaders throughout China (PRC) and South East Asia in areas of telemedicine and teleradiology, healthcare informatics and tele-education.

Since 1996, he has Co-directed InHouse Radiology Medical Group, Inc. and InHouse Radiology Medical Management, LLC., niche providers of tele-radiology services to clinicians in private offices performing digital diagnostic imaging. He previously served as Senior Attending Surgeon in the Division of Neurological Surgery at Cedars-Sinai Medical Center in Los Angeles, California, and as Vice Chairman in the Division of Neurological Surgery. He also served as Senior Consultant in Neurological Surgery at the City of Hope National Medical Center inDuarte, California.

At that time, Dr. Saunders served as Chief of Neurological Surgery, Century City Hospital, and as Chief of Neurological Surgery and Co-Director of the Comprehensive Spine Center at Midway Hospital in Los Angeles. He served as a Clinical Instructor at UCLA School of Medicine, Department of Neurological Surgery, and Wadsworth Veterans Administration Hospital.